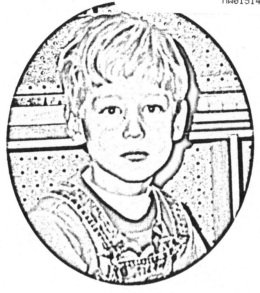

# TREASURES
# OF
# DARKNESS

*Unwrapping the Gift of Autism*

SALLY BRENDEN

Unless otherwise noted, Scripture quotations are taken from the *Holy Bible*, New Living Translation (NLT). © 1996. Used by permission of Tyndale House Publishers, Inc., Wheaton, Illinois 60189. All rights reserved.

Other Scripture references are from the following sources: Holy Bible, New International Version®, NIV® (NIV). © 1973,1978, 1984 by Biblica Inc.™ Used by permission of Zondervan. All rights reserved worldwide. New King James Version®. © 1982 by Thomas Nelson, Inc. Used by permission. All rights reserved. King James Version (KJV).

Graphic Design by Stefanie Brenden and Karen's Koncepts

# Table of Contents

# DEDICATION

Dedicated to my Beloved Children

Matthew

Chad

&

Stefanie

# ACKNOWLEDGMENTS

There are loved ones who have chosen to look at Chad through the lens of the heart. They have walked along side me, discovering the great treasure that is Chad. Thank you.

Chad's father Mel, his brother Matthew, sister Stefanie, and my "almost son" Scott Abel have loved Chad well. I could not have survived without my mom, Delight Nelson, now with Jesus. There are aunts and uncles and cousins who love Chad; dear friends and colleagues, also.

I gratefully acknowledge Amy Eickhoff for her ministry of The Rock, created for young adults including Chad, the dear Ellgen family, and Larry Oseid, who greets and shakes hands with Chad at church every Sunday. Also, Mark Rostad, for his warm acceptance of Chad and the tradition of choosing to celebrate their mutual birthday at Red Lobster.

I wish to acknowledge the loving contributions of teachers and educational staff, especially Theresa Maas, Annemarie Loehning, Dan Blaisdell, Amy Johnson, Denise Weekley, Vicki Zager and Sue Paasch. Chad's counselor, Deb Lalley, and social workers Vickie Waytashek and Margot Lorsung have helped us navigate difficult waters.

Adding richness to Chad's life are professionals from community based agencies providing services, Kristine Hollingsworth standing out as the most awesome advocate ever, and his beautiful and precious friends on his work crew and in The Rock.

Thank you to Brad and Ann Hanson, and the caring staff and precious housemates at ABH Homes, Chad's new "family". Finding you was a truly a gift from God.

I thank my precious son, Chad, for accepting his mission as being God's James Bond. Chad, living with you is like living with Jesus. Thank you.

And most of all, I acknowledge my dependence upon my dear Savior for wisdom and strength to raise Chad, for the privilege of being his mother, and for the certain hope of spending eternity with my son.

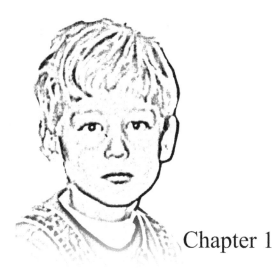

# Chapter 1

# *"I Could Live in Sheboygan"*

"You know, Mom!" twelve year Chad announced excitedly, "When I grow up, I could live in Paris! New York! Los Angeles! Florida! Chicago! I could live in Sheboygan!!"

Sheboygan?

Yes, Sheboygan!

Welcome to the world of autism!

Perhaps you have read Emily Perl Kingsley's classic "Welcome to Holland"[1], a poignant perspective on discovering your child has a disability and that your life has taken an unplanned detour to a "foreign country." She uses the rich imagery of pregnancy as planning an exciting vacation trip to Italy, and upon de-boarding your flight finding out you have actually landed in Holland. You have arrived at a location you neither planned nor wanted to visit. But that is where you are and where you will spend your trip. Wise the person who stops

1

focusing on the loss of Italy and chooses to see the unique beauty and treasure of Holland.

While this spin on a child with a disability is beautiful and true in many respects, I could never totally relate to it. Because living with autism is far from living in Holland.

Living with autism is one day having a visitor from the most remote and primitive village show up on your doorstep.

Intellectually, you may believe it is an enriching experience to have someone from another culture become part of your family.

You may even come to bond with this person before he returns to his home, perhaps feeling gratification that you could reach out and do something for the poor unfortunate and under privileged person.

But if on this day, this same *uninvited* visitor appears at your door with adoption papers naming you as parent, and moves in as a permanent member of the family, everything you know intellectually vanishes. So does the shallow bonding. If you think you can align the two vastly different cultures into any semblance of a fit, you are in for a rude awakening.

Let me tell you what it is like when autism invades the sanctity of your home.

Suddenly there is a visitor in your home that you did not invite. And he plans to stay the rest of his life. And with him, he brings his constant companion, chronic sorrow.

Kiss any dreams of a fairy tale life you had cherished goodbye.

Everything about your visitor is different, starting with very basic survival issues - food and sleep. Even these are challenges. His food choices are different. His body clock is different. His sleep patterns are different. He communicates differently to put it mildly. He may not be able to tell you he's sick. He needs your constant protection and guidance. His behavior is unpredictable. His activities are peculiar; his ideas often bizarre. He obsesses over strange things.

Your other kids wonder why he is so unusual, and why he gets so much of your attention. It drives you crazy when he gets angry or sad or nervous and you can't reason with him and help him. You become exhausted trying to find a way to communicate with his illogical thought patterns. You must learn to predict behavior and manage environments several steps in advance to head off some of the inescapable problems. Everyone who meets him wonders why he is different and looks at you, some with pity, some with disgust, and those who also have had similar visitors come unexpectedly to live with them, with love and understanding.

Your new family member can never truly become acculturated to this new environment. He was not made for the fast paced, high pressured,competitive, dog-eat-dog global society that we exist in. And to force him to fit in, to become like you, will destroy your visitor.

If you both make changes and adaptations, you can forge a workable relationship. Plan on being the one to do most of the changing and adapting as this is almost impossible for your visitor.

There is one thing you must understand. You can never fully enter each other's worlds. Rather than change his world, you seek to understand him by entering his.

You move to "Sheboygan".

Why Sheboygan? There is no logical answer. An autistic mind works in its own way. And to Chad, Sheboygan holds every bit the same charm as the Louvre, the Eiffel Tower, Disney World and the Statue of Liberty.

When Chad was a preschooler, we knew his world wasn't the same as ours. So we moved with him to "Sheboygan". And with the move, began an unimagined life.

3

And in a paradox that only God could engineer, it became the life I would have chosen.

How long has it been since you went on a treasure hunt? Come with me. We're headed to "Sheboygan".

Did I mention there is no map?

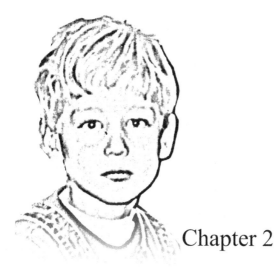

## Chapter 2

# *"A Problem Has Arrived"*

I knew in an instant something was wrong. His breathing changed. His movements trying to get comfy under his covers were different. Mothers sense those things. Dog tired from no sleep and five hours until the alarm would go off, I drug myself out of bed and into Chad's bedroom. For the nth time since he'd been put to bed two hours before. As I walked toward him he announced predictably, "A problem has arrived."

I had no clue a problem had arrived when a precious seven pound boy was put in my arms on 21 January 1987. There was nothing unusual about the pregnancy. Aside from horrendous morning sickness, which was my norm, everything was fine. After the traumatic and life threatening experience with my first child, Matthew, it was a given from day one that Chad would be an elective C-section. I had no complications, no problems. There was also nothing unusual about his early development. No red flags. Matt had done everything early, speaking and walking at barely eight months, and I accepted Chad's little slower pace as perfectly normal. He was crawling by six and one half months, speaking his first word at eight months and walking by eleven months.

He was cuddly, loved to be held and interacted with others. My sister Meg's most vivid early memory of Chad was how unusually cuddly he was.

At age two, baby sister Stefanie was added to the family. I truly had not noticed anything of concern at this time. On his second birthday, I wrote this in his baby book:

> You are a delightful little person. You talk quite a bit, though not elaborately. Shorter sentences like, "Mama, read, please." You love to be read to, love to color, watch Sesame Street, play basketball, play with minnows and with Matthew's tackle box. You love to be outside and go to Grandma Nelson's or Grandma Brenden's. You love to be held and cuddled and want "tunes" at bedtime.

Within the next year, I began to see little things that caught my attention.

- He colored everything black.
- He never asked "why?" questions.
- He had a phenomenal visual memory. McDonalds had a huge display board of the Dick Tracy characters and after the first time he saw it, he knew every character and a matching characteristic. (I got the display from the manager when the promotion ended and it was Chad's favorite possession.) You could not trick him on Lips Manlis or Pruneface or Big Boy Caprice. He was fixated with brand names of toilet stools and became very frustrated if I couldn't report instantly from memory the brand at every business establishment we had visited even once.
- He started putting a blanket or towel around his shoulders to wear as a cape.
- He started gathering objects, the same ones all the time, and put them on an easy chair or in the corner of the living room where he "hung out".
- A picture shows him neatly arranging all the clothes from his

dresser on the kitchen floor.

- A studio Christmas picture of the kids when Chad was not quite three shows a beautiful smiley blonde boy but on close observation Matthew and Stefanie are looking into the camera and Chad's eyes are turned away.
- He had strange interests such as scouting for road kill. I kid you not.

I thought of autism and had even said to my husband from time to time, "That's autistic behavior" but I thought of autism as the far end of the spectrum and comforted myself that it couldn't be. While not as verbal, he had no problem communicating and he was happy, cuddly and smart.

Yet, looking back, it was all there, though not full blown, as evidenced by my entry in his baby book on his third birthday.

> You are talking a lot. Good words-"am frackers" (graham crackers), "frig-a-frator" (refrigerator). You use many Swedish words. You are polite. "Tank you. Sorry. Excuse me. Please." You can amuse yourself well. You like to pretend you're Batman and often have a baby sheet over your shoulder and a cowboy hat on your head. You drag sheets all over the floor and have a regular routine. You like movies (Willie Wonka, Pee Wee Christmas, Winnie the Pooh) and TV (Reading Rainbow, Mr. Rogers, Shining Time Station).

> You enjoy painting very much and painting shows on TV are your favorites. You like to use just one color–usually a dark color. You color, use chalk and draw. You like reading your books. You like dogs–especially Aunty Meg's dog and proudly tell us "Sandra obeys Chad". Your speech is cute–not elaborate, but fun. "That terrible bird went poop on Mama's car. Terrible bad."

When he was almost four my Christmas letter read:

> Chad is quiet, plays well alone and loves to listen to music. Unfortunately he enjoys Charlie Rich. He was really into Dick Tracy this summer and would ask passersby "Who's your favorite criminal?" This fall he got into the political campaigns

and memorized most of the signs. He even prayed for the candidates—a practice we highly encouraged.

The next year's Christmas letter updated Chad's life at age five:
Chad has advanced from scouting road kill to culinary pursuits. Specialties include kosher dill pickles and cold cereal sandwiches and banana juice.

(Lest you think I am a respecter of persons, it's not like the rest of the family look normal. Stefanie now believes she's a cat. The upside is that it has motivated her to use a litter box. Matt's greatest interest is following his Daddy crawling through muddy cornfields on his belly after geese.)

There is one last entry in his baby book on his sixth birthday.
You started Learning Readiness three days a week along with one day of Early Childhood. You seem to like it. Your teacher is Theresa Maas. You like playing electronic games, your musical instruments, and art work like making hats and drawing people. You are printing your letters. You like riding your bike at the park and pretending outside. You have imaginary stores: a candy store, a restaurant, a toy store. You and Stefanie argue and tease; she teases and you moan. You love fellowship at night. You are very cuddly and affectionate then. You like books. You are very into Bible stories. Sisera, Jeremiah, Solomon and Zacharias are favorites.

~

Looking back, at about age three he began to go inward. Although I knew nothing of interventions strategies, God granted me wisdom. Endless times throughout the day I would touch him, look him in the eye and make him respond. He stayed in our world. I have since learned that in just a short amount of time at this critical period an autistic child can go inward and be lost.

Amazingly, along with the serious challenge of keeping Chad in our world, I recall mainly dealing with the situation in such an exhausting life by finding the humor in the situation.

When he was about three and one half, I wrote the following story:

## Encouraging Kids Creativity or Fred Sanford Rides Again

*Child experts are supposed to know what they are talking about.*

*They claim that if you want your children to develop good self concepts, which, of course all of us inadequate parents want for our kids, you need to provide opportunities for them to play creatively and explore the things they enjoy.*

*Sounds great on the surface but what if the ghost of Fred Sanford lurks within your three year old?*

*My first son's interests were almost within the normal range on the Bell Curve. Not so with number two. Let me just say his favorite outdoor activity is seeking out fresh road kill. Playing indoors is no problem either. He can amuse himself for hours creating his own little kingdom of LaLa Land in our living room.*

*Now our house is small; we're not talking sprawling hacienda. The living room is little as in there-is-room-for-essentials-only-and-not-one-item-of-clutter.*

*Tell that to Chad.*

*The first thing he drags out in the morning long before sunrise is his pillow and pink blanket which some dear soul made for baby sister Stefanie but Chad immediately confiscated for his own usage. Then out of the linen closet come the sheets. Fitted sheets, top sheets, crib sheets. And towels: beach towels, bath towels, hand towels, dish towels; wet towels, dry towels, musty towels; orange towels, gold towels, brown towels, plaid towels, and heaven forbid if the towel with the zoo animals is missing.*

*Next are all the belts in the house and Daddy's old ties which were on their way to the Salvation Army but, again, were appropriated for Chad's creative pleasure.*

9

*Then it's to his dresser to haul all his shirts and sweaters to the living room. His underwear and pants drawers are left undisturbed.*

*We've only just begun. Next the kitchen is raided. He needs two glass containers of instant coffee, two of instant tea and one jar of instant orange drink. And spices-dry mustard, cinnamon, chili powder and cream of tarter are musts (don't even think of trying to trick him and give substitutes). And the baking powder with the Native American chief.*

*This is just the beginning of his foray into the kitchen. Tongs, spatulas, measuring spoons, a chopstick (one is forever lost), and wooden spoons. Pots and pans, a stove top coffee pot and stainless steel and plastic mixing bowls to wear on his head are quickly hauled to his cache in the living room. The colander is his favorite hat. He even tried to wear it to church but his father quickly put the kibosh on that. I thought nothing of it. I have no recollection of a time in my life since I became a mother that I possessed either pride or dignity.*

*There's more, so much more starting with all the pencils in the house, but not pens, markers or crayons. Bibles, VCR tapes taken out of the boxes, all my piano books long devoid of covers and all seven books in the Chronicles of Narnia series. Stuffed animals, blocks, toy soldiers, card games, and tidbits from favorite board games. His brother's tackle box with plastic worms, salamanders and spinner baits, opened, of course, and contents emptied. And our meager record collection which stands at about eight, including "My Name is Zoom and I Live on the Moon" (from a cereal box offer), all records being removed from their respective jackets.*

*Chad puts all he can into one easy chair. The rest of the treasures are in a heap next to the chair under a floor lamp.*

*Did I mention books, color books, hand held electronic games, Daddy's fishing magazines, Christmas and birthday cards he fancies, and his brother's lunch box?*

*I mustn't omit the winter clothing which is gathered year round: snow pants, jacket, boots, hats, mittens; my unsightly green rubber hunting boots; and all the gloves in the household, especially the one-of-a-pair kinds.*

*The most precious items of all are his Dick Tracy, Batman and Elvis item including slates, color books, pictures, boxes and bags. Anything to do with these characters is kept close at hand day and night. And any pictures of Abe Lincoln and George "Washingmachine".*

*To collect all of this requires strength. So nourishment is brought in. Chips, nachos and crackers are favorites. He isn't fussy though he does refuse anything that doesn't leave crumbs. To this standard list, various new items are added daily as the spirit moves.Amazingly in the midst of all his treasures he knows just when one item is missing and will wail bitterly, "Itchy (or Shoulders or fill-in-the-blank) is missing!"*

*To which I respond consolingly, "Chad, it IS possible that a one inch object could be momentarily misplaced."*

*Yes, there are times when I can't see the living room carpet that I question the wisdom of the child experts with their easily doled out advice on letting Freddy Sanford use his imagination.*

*But even if they are dead wrong I have nothing to lose.*

*The living room is still the cleanest room in my house!*

~

Admittedly, I exaggerate a tad. (Blame it on genetics, proof being an elderly maternal aunt winning Honorable Mention in the Burlington Liars Contest.) But just a tad.

This was the Beginning. It was all too apparent that indeed "A Problem *Had* Arrived."

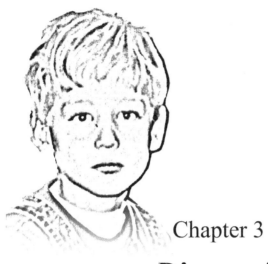

## Chapter 3

# *Diagnosis*

"There's something terribly wrong with your child. Pervasive Developmental Disorder. You should have started something a long time ago."

I was unprepared for the sudden onslaught of words. Just words, but such words, thrown in my face, in that tone of voice; words that in an instant turned my little world upside down. And in the presence of my four year old son!

"Who do you think you are and what do you think you're doing?" I angrily replied. "My son is here. He can hear, you know," my instinct to protect my son suddenly shifting into overdrive.

Knowing something was amiss, and knowing enough of autism to believe that was the most likely scenario, I had arranged for the only pediatrician at our clinic to meet with Chad. She had spent a short time with him, attempting to engage him in several activities with limited success. Pushed beyond his limit, Chad was lying on the floor.

My parenthood attacked, my world spinning, my only goal was to get Chad and I away from that awful person and out of that terrible room as fast as I could.

"You may be right." I said, "But how you have just treated us was inexcusable. We won't be back."

We gingerly made our way through the mine fields of the next four years. I called our school district and got involved with Early Childhood Special Education that fall. The next year he went to a combination pre-kindergarten/early childhood program, then on to kindergarten and into the first grade.

The school personnel were wonderful. They often questioned the diagnosis because for a "high functioning" autistic child, many times there is interfacing with normalcy. But none of us ever questioned there were significant issues and they would cry with me as we sat on the living room floor during home visits and at conferences.

~

The school needed a diagnosis by the time Chad was seven to continue Special Education services. We asked our family doctor for a referral. Incidentally, I had taken Chad to him in the intervening years and he strongly questioned the diagnosis of his colleague, encouraging us to keep doing exactly what we were doing.

Armed with Psalm 112:7-8, we headed down to the appointment in Minneapolis.

> They do not fear bad news; they confidently trust the Lord to care for them. They are confident and fearless …..

Chad spent time with a Clinical Psychologist and a Developmental/ Behavioral Pediatrician.

Three weeks later we went back for the results.

The diagnosis:
"Mild autistic disorder with associated sensory motor
integration difficulties"

The diagnosis was formal. The prognosis was for a lifetime. There was no comfort in the descriptor "mild".

I am well aware that there are stories about children who have miraculously emerged from the dark cocoon of autism. Of parents who were given the gift of helping set them free. There are stories of profoundly autistic children who have emerged into brilliant and social adults, totally devoid of any vestige of autism.

But they are rare, very rare.

And, what is very noticeable to me is that most are not shared from the viewpoint of factoring in Jesus and His plan.

Where does God fit in to the diagnosis? Am I supposed to accept, even embrace autism? Or, should I be consumed with the desire to change the prognosis?

~

I know God could intervene. It would be nothing for the Creator and Controller of the Universe with every molecule at His command to lift Chad from autism in the twinkling of an eye. God can, but He usually doesn't. I believe God can heal people terminally ill with cancer, yet I personally have never seen this happen. The many that I have known, to the very last one, have not been healed. They were handed the gift of an unwanted treasure. But rather than embracing this gift, many devoted their energies toward changing the prognosis, rather than accepting God's call to an unwanted ministry in their lives.

For me, it is the same with autism. Could it be a gift in disguise? Hidden treasures and secret riches may come packaged in the brown wrapping paper of autism. Should they be rejected? Or, like any treasure and riches, should they be valued and yes, even embraced?

My inner conviction, in our situation, is to accept Chad unconditionally as he is, to commit him totally to God and to go on. Yes, early on I asked God to heal. But I didn't demand. For as difficult as autism is, and at times it is unbearable, my biggest fear is the possibility that God would grant my request at great expense only eternity would reveal.

> And He gave them their request, but sent leanness into their soul. (Psalm 106:15 NKJV)

What a far greater tragedy than autism!

My whole life has been one of preparation for a child with special needs.

There are some things you just know. Like Mary you ponder them in your heart and when the time comes you say, "I've always known." There is quiet serenity of the heart. A "Be it done unto me according to Thy Word" contract where all you say to God is "Yes!"

~

I have always known that if I had children there would be some special challenges. Each time one was born, I was surprised that there were no visible indications as to what these challenges might be *because I knew*.

Ever since childhood something in my spirit has risen up every time I heard the following conversation.

> "Oh, so you're expecting a little one! Are you hoping for a boy or girl?"

> (You know the bottled response.)
> "It doesn't matter--AS LONG AS IT'S HEALTHY."

> And I would say, "So if it's not healthy, you don't want it?" And in my heart, even as a child, I would say, "God, I'll take the ones that someone else doesn't think are as good."

16

What do I want for my children? What is my ultimate goal for my children? It has nothing to do with social skills, brilliance, accomplishments, power, prestige, talent, fame, or their making me look great as a parent.

I made only one request regarding any child I would ever have: that they would spend eternity with Jesus. Nothing else. No conditions. Only eternity with Jesus. If they could hear, see, walk, think, use the bathroom independently - such nonessentials would only be God's gifts.

God has given Chad and me, by default, a ministry beyond description in his autism. I cannot share anything about who he is without sharing Jesus. And the curious thing is that no one ever has been offended. That's a gift. It is an open door. It is a ministry I would not have asked for, perhaps one I would have determinedly avoided, but it is truly an open door.

Many of us faith-based parents theoretically give our children back to God in some sort of dedication ceremony, formal or informal, when they are young. It may be a dedication, a baptism. We tell God that the child is really His and we are raising the child for Him. Theoretically, we surrender all rights to God to use this child as He pleases. Theoretically, there are no strings attached.

But when we are hit with the diagnosis, the illness and the challenges we say, "No, God, that's not what I meant. You can't do that with *my* child. You need to do it *my* way."

Yet our hearts burn for the lost and we tell God in sincerity we would give our very lives for these dear ones to come to Him. So He provides an open door where God's grace is displayed and where the lost can see Him, and we say "No, God, not at the expense of my child. That's where I draw the line."

And we miss the big plan and picture with our myopic vision.

It's not like God is asking us to go through something He hasn't. He did not withhold suffering from His Son. His Son came and for thirty three years lived in a world that didn't fit him either. Everything about Him was different. But His suffering gave me Life. God could have stepped in and made everything all comfortable and easy for Jesus. But then there would have been no Calvary. And then there would have been no Hope.

God has the big picture in mind. His ways are not our ways.
> "My thoughts are completely different from yours", says the Lord. "And my ways are far beyond anything you could imagine. For just as the heavens are higher than the earth, so are my ways higher than your ways and my thoughts higher than your thoughts." (Isaiah 55:8- 9)

~

I have always been a Big Picture person. Perhaps that is why it is easier for me to accept autism than it is for many other people. Even I can see how God can take Chad, my precious little Picnic Basket of "five loaves and two fishes," bless him, multiply him, and feed hungry people.

Chad's love for Jesus has touched many. Would more be touched by his healing? Only God knows. So I leave it in His hands.

And I embrace autism, seeking primarily not to change, but to find the secret riches of hidden places and the treasures of darkness as I explore God's wonderful plan for my son and me in this terribly difficult adventure, asking only that God walk before us.

> **I will give you the treasures of darkness, riches stored in secret places**…. (Isaiah 45:3a NIV)

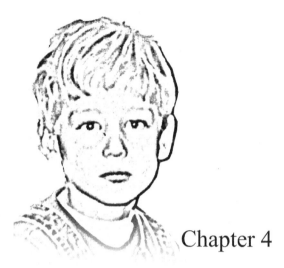

## Chapter 4

# *"Just the Facts, Ma'am"*

Those of us Baby Boomers who grew up in the days of the popular TV show "Dragnet" remember one statement made all too popular by Sgt. Joe Friday: "Just the facts, Ma'am!"

At times it is sage advice and not just for the Baby Boomers.

Autism is an intriguing mystery. When Chad was young, my idea of an autistic child was that of a baby never wanting to be held, a small child spending his day sitting in a corner spinning objects and writing the same peculiar phrase over and over, or the adult savant who could recite every weather fact for Tucumcari, New Mexico on October 13, 1964.

I rather hate facts. Facts are so detached; so hard, cold, clinical, sobering and confining. There's always so much more to the picture than the facts.

Admittedly it is the necessary place to begin. And with my son, facts regarding autism must be faced and accepted.

I don't like the facts. I want to fight them. Change them. Pretend they're not true. Sugarcoat them to make them easier to swallow. I want them less threatening, less scary, and certainly not for a lifetime.

I could give you all the facts of autism but I won't because your life is full of your own facts. They are different than mine, but they are there. In your face, embedded in your life, for none of us is exempt from ugly and unwanted facts.

Your facts aren't any easier to face than mine. And, like me, you want to fight them. Change them. Pretend they're not true. Make them easier to swallow, less threatening, less scary, and certainly not for a lifetime.

Facts! Yes, we often have to begin with them. But we don't have to be blown away by them.

They are only part of the picture! Mercifully, a small part of the picture!

I have words of encouragement for you.

Actually, two words.

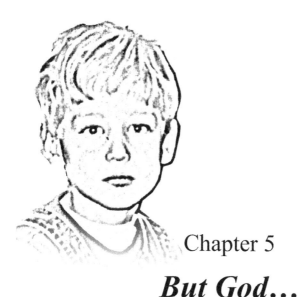

Chapter 5

# *But God...*

But God...

My favorite words in the Bible.

Two words harnessing the power of the entire universe and offering an eternal perspective to every life experience. Two words promising God's provision for every situation. Two words allowing me a glimpse into His perfect plan and purpose for my life, for my son's life, for your life.

I have never faced a challenge in life but that these two words have had the power to revolutionize the experience.

Hungry for hope? Starving for something to strengthen you for your journey into unwanted facts? Pull up a chair at the table of God's Word. He has a feast waiting just for you! I'll be your server. What beverage would you like? Coffee? Tea? Milk? Lemonade? Diet soda?

We'll start with an appetizer. I have made two words stand out to whet your appetite.

> My health may fail, and my spirit may grow weak, BUT GOD remains the strength of my heart; he is mine forever. (Psalm 73:26)

> You intended to harm me, BUT GOD intended it for good to accomplish what is now being done… (Genesis 50:20 NIV)

Help yourself to as many entrees as you wish.

> BUT GOD showed his great love for us by sending Christ to die for us while we were still sinners. (Romans 5:8)

> BUT GOD is so rich in mercy, and he loved us so very much, that even while we were dead because of our sins, he gave us life when he raised Christ from the dead. (Ephesians 2:4-5)

> Jesus looked at them intently and said, "Humanly speaking, it is impossible, BUT with GOD everything is possible." (Matthew 19:26)

> BUT my GOD shall supply all your need according to his riches in glory by Christ Jesus. (Philippians 4:19 KJV)

> These sons of Jacob were very jealous of their brother Joseph, and they sold him to be a slave in Egypt. BUT GOD was with him and delivered him from his anguish. And God gave him favor… (Acts 7: 9-10a)

May I bring you a refill on your drink?

> Do not be afraid! Don't be discouraged by this mighty army, for the battle is not yours, BUT GOD's. (2 Chronicles 20:15b)

> BUT GOD did listen! He paid attention to my prayer. (Psalm 66:19)

I hope you've saved room for dessert!!

> "No eye has seen, no ear has heard, no mind has conceived what God has prepared for those who love him" -- BUT GOD has revealed it to us by his Spirit. (1 Corinthians 2:9-10 NIV) BUT GOD will redeem my life from the grave; he will surely take me to himself. (Psalm 49:15 NIV)

Did you fill up? If you didn't, there's much more on the menu that I could recommend.

But God.

When you need a snack or a five course meal, come back again. There's all you can eat and it's calorie-free!

By the way, there is no charge for your meal. Your Father picked up the tab.

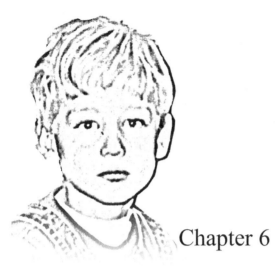

Chapter 6

# *The Moment*

I have never felt such pain. I have never felt a greater love.

It was a school morning in May. Chad was ten years old. All the pressure of coping, adapting and learning had caught up with him. His resources were depleted. He was empty.

Several weeks before he had thrown up on the way to the bus stop. He hadn't spoken of being ill, of dreading school. He got up, dressed, and headed out the door without complaint. And heaved his little guts out.

I brought him in hoping it was the flu, but knowing it wasn't. He was fine the rest of the day. That evening he asked me if he was sick like that again would he have to go to school. I said, "Chad, you're not really sick with the flu. You're sick because you're nervous and worried and it's so hard to cope at school. If it happens again, you can come in the house and wait until you stop throwing up and then Mama will take you to school."

Then came the morning in May. Once again, between the kitchen door and the approaching bus, without warning, Chad got sick.

I had never discussed autism with him. We had danced around the subject. He knew he was different. He knew some things were hard for him and that was the way God had made him. But I had never given it a name.

I was asked from time to time if I had told him. I said, "No, the time hasn't come. When it does, I'll know, and then I'll tell him."

His younger sister, Stefanie, went on to the bus stop alone. I took Chad back in the house, wrapped him in a comforter and held him. Almost immediately he was fine.

About an hour later I told him that I was going to take him to school. He became unglued. "But Mom, I can't go to school! It's already started. I'll be late!"

I explained that was no big deal. I'd take him and explain everything to the teacher.

"NO! I can't go!" he persisted, signs of approaching hysteria mounting. Firmly and calmly I said, "Chad, you have to go to school."

Tears flowed, his little body shook and he begged, "But Mom, I CAN'T GO. I NEED THIS FOR MY LIFE!"

That is autism speaking. He seldom states this, but when he does, it truly means he needs it for his life.

The Moment had come. We were alone and it was the time.

"Chad," I said, "Mama has something very important to tell you."

He sat on the arm of the living room recliner, next to me, listening attentively, sensing the urgency of what I was about to say. The conversation is forever etched in my memory.

"Chad, the reason you threw up on the way to the bus was not because you were sick with something like the flu. I think your body got sick because you were worried and nervous about school. Do you think that might have been what happened?"

"Maybe."

"It's okay that you get worried and nervous about school. That's the way God made you and it's okay. God made you very special, Chad. There's a lot of things that are hard for you and make you worried and nervous. Isn't that right?"

"I guess so."

"There's a name for the way God made you, Chad. It's autistic. Can you say autistic?"

"Autistic."

"That's right. Autistic. When people are autistic they worry more than other people. It's harder to cope with life. Things can make them nervous and afraid. Do you think you get nervous and worry and have trouble coping?"

"Probably."

"That's okay. That's the way God made you and God made you just the way He wanted you. He made you autistic and that's just the way you're supposed to be. Everybody has issues, things that are hard for them. Some people are blind. What can't they do?"

"See."

"Some people are in wheelchairs. What might they not be able to do?"

"To walk?"

"Yes, that's one reason people are in wheelchairs. There's a lot of things Mama can't do. I drop everything and I'm a terrible singer. Matt and Stefanie have things that are hard for them, too, but they aren't autistic. Neither is Daddy."

"Chad, when people are autistic, like you, some things are especially hard for them. It's harder to make friends. You play differently and like different things. And sometimes you'd just rather be alone, wouldn't you?"

"Probably."

"And school is hard, isn't it? Paying attention and listening all day and learning everything. That's really hard for autistic children. And noises and big noisy groups of people and things like basketball games can be too loud and scary, can't they?"

(Head nod.)

"Now I want to tell you the most important thing. You won't always be autistic. When you get to heaven, everything will be perfect. You'll never worry. You'll never be afraid. You'll have all the friends you want. You love Jesus, don't you Chad?"

"YES, I LOVE JESUS!"

"I know, Babe, and that's all that matters. Nothing else matters in the whole world except that you love Jesus. And I know you do, Chad. I think you must be Jesus' favorite little boy in the whole universe."

"And He loves you. And He'll always be with you. If Mama could take away your autism, I would. But I can't. If Mama could make everything right so you'd never worry or be afraid or nervous, I would. But I can't."

"You will always be autistic until you get to heaven. It will be hard, Chad. Mama and Daddy can't change that. We'll always do everything we can to help you and try to make it so you aren't too afraid or worried. But we can't make everything okay."

"Mama, why are you crying?"

"Because I love you so much Chad."

"Remember Jesus is always with you. And when things are hard and you're afraid or you can't cope, just tell Jesus in your mind and He'll help you because He loves you more than anyone in the universe."

"Do you understand what Mama's telling you, Chad?"

"Don't cry so hard Mama."

"I can't help it, Chad. I love you so much."

"Do you have any questions, Chad, or anything you want to tell Mama?"

(Head shake as he looks away to break the intimacy.)

"Okay. Do you need to stay home the rest of the day and be with Mama and think about the important things we talked about?"

"Yes. And I'll go to school tomorrow."

"That sounds like a good plan, Sweetheart. I love you!"

"I love you, too, Mom."

Love and pain, in equal measure, filled me, threatening to consume me. And then Hope rushed in and flooded my spirit. Hope for Chad! Hope for me! Hope because eternity shouts at the end of the equation.

If autism cannot be put in light of eternity, there is no hope for Chad. All the attempts to make autism palatable are a crock. It is all empty talk. Either God knows what He's doing, or disabilities are a cosmic joke. If I cannot explain autism to Chad in light of eternity, I have nothing to give him as a foundation, no lifeline to throw out. I am an empty person offering him nothing, giving him an empty plate with nothing on it to sustain and nourish him.

Without Jesus as a base, there are no words of hope at the Moment of Truth. But with Jesus, what a different story!

I re-wrapped Chad in his comforter, got one for myself and we laid in the living room, I on the couch, Chad snuggled next to me on the floor, holding my hand. And wasted from the enormity of the experience, we both slept for 3 hours.

It was 9 A.M.

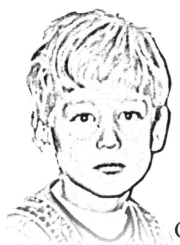

Chapter 7

# *Born to Love God*

There was one thing that deeply troubled me when I suspected Chad was autistic. If he couldn't relate to people, how would be he able to relate to God?

An encouraging thing happened as I pondered this. There was an article in our local paper about a sixteen year old autistic young man.[2] Severely autistic, he had lost his speech and been put into a home for autistic children at age five because of his violent behavior. His family brought him home at age ten, because, according to his father, they realized God had given him to them for a reason, and they'd never regretted the decision.

At age sixteen, he learned to communicate using facilitated communication. Using his computer to respond to the questions of the reporter in two interviews, the young man's comments pierced my heart.

When asked what he wanted to do in the future, he wrote that wanted to preach the Gospel to lost people. He wrote that he had learned the

Gospel from God and that God talks to him out loud and tells him that He loves him and it will be OK.

Using his facilitated communication, he wrote that it was hard to be autistic and that he wanted to talk but was locked inside his body which was like a prison. He added that wanted to write, like the Apostle Paul who was in prison and wrote to help others.

When asked what he most wanted people to know, this wise young man responded that he loved God and he loved people and that he was learning to live life the way God wanted him to live.

My prayer for Chad became, not that God would heal, but that He would reveal. That Chad might know God with every fiber of his being.

I recalled the story attributed to Helen Keller who, upon learning God's name, said she had always known Him. She just hadn't known His name.[3]

And my heart cried out to God many times over the years, "Reveal Yourself to my son."

God has honored my prayer. Chad has an unusual love and heart for God.

I remember the first time he took communion. He had observed but never requested to participate. One Sunday, when he was about seven, communion was to be served. He said, "Mom, can I take it?"

I have always believed little ones who love Jesus have an equal right to sit at God's table, even though they can't digest the same foods and their manners may be a bit sloppy.

"Communion is for anyone, old or young, who loves Jesus and has Jesus living in their heart, Chad," I said. "Do you love Jesus and have Jesus in your heart?"

"Yes, Mom, YOU KNOW I LOVE JESUS." He looked shocked that I'd even ask.

"Then you may, Sweetheart," I said. And I watched as with reverence his little fingers picked up the tiny cracker and held the little cup of grape juice and was certain he knew more of the meaning of communion than most adults.

And when I tucked him in that night, he said, "Today was the best day of my life. I loved communion. And I love Jesus."

One summer day, when he was ten, he came up to me as I was working in the kitchen and said, "I know why I was born."

Knowing I was about to hear something profound, I stopped, put him on my lap and said, "Tell me, Chad, why were you born?"

"I was born to love God," said my little blonde angel.

Through tears I held him close and said, "You're so right, Chad. You were born to love God. That's all--just to love God." And he grabbed his ever present jump rope and went back outside to play.

> Then Jesus prayed this prayer: "O Father, Lord of heaven and earth, thank you for hiding the truth from those who think themselves so wise and clever, and for revealing it to the childlike." (Matthew 11:25)

We were all born to love God.

But how few of us know.

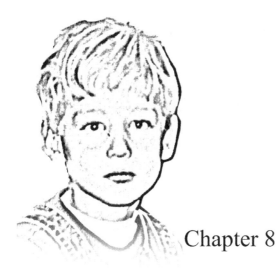

Chapter 8

# *A Day in the Life*

Our days are like any other family. School. Work. Shopping. Doctor appointments. Driver's Training. But autism makes it more than school, work, shopping, doctor appointments, and driver's training.

I write about a day in our life. Yesterday.

Because I had everything done the night before, I sleep in until almost 5 a.m. This is my time alone. Coffee in the living room watching the worship videos, thinking, reading, praying. Alone and quiet. I get ready for work and have a bowl of cold cereal.

Chad and Stefanie get up at 6:15. I wrap them both in comforters and bring them to the couch to wake up. They watch morning cartoons. Stefanie will drink cocoa and have a bite to eat. I work with Chad for the next forty five minutes trying to get him to drink a few swallows of water. He won't eat. He also won't eat much at school; maybe juice at juice break. I send snacks-fruit snacks, crackers, favorite juices - anything he picks out at the store that he thinks he would eat at school.

35

When he goes for individual help, he always brings a snack so we can get food in him. He will drink a few swallows of mineral water at lunch in the lunchroom. No more. Maybe he will have a piece of candy if he is lucky enough to win one at multiplication bingo.

He has lost thirteen pounds in the past year. The doctor feels it is stress related and not physical. His food patterns are erratic. The previous year, he had gotten too heavy, eating almost nonstop from the time he got home from school. Many times before bed he would eat three or four dishes of cold cereal. During the summer I had worked to be sure he ate a bit more nutritiously and took him swimming every day. Food battles are not to be chosen during the school year; school is its own major battle. So I was happy to see him slimming down. But one day in the fall I noticed his face was getting drawn and his weight loss, gradual to that point, became a concern. By great vigilance I have been able to keep him at his present weight for the past three months - no gain, but no loss.

It is 6:52; time to brush teeth and dress for school. I have the clothes all lying by the living room heat vents so they are toasty. The stress of the morning makes Chad's little body just shake from the chill and fear. We pray and head out for school at 7:10. We make sure we do everything by the clock.

This year I started taking the kids to school. Sometimes Stefanie rides the bus. Chad had always been great at going on the bus both to and from school until this year. This fall he started a new school. Now he and Stefanie go to different schools. One of the first days of school, after Stefanie got off, he was apparently sitting near the back of the bus. The kids are one of the last on and the bus is crowded. Until this year, I had always made arrangements for a front seat to be saved for Chad, but somehow he ended up near the back. He told me the following story when he came home.

"I had a terrible time on the bus this morning. Some of the kids started asking me questions and laughed at my answers and kept asking more and laughing at the answers and then they said, 'Chad, you don't know anything' and I said 'Yes, I do, I know lots of things' and they really hurt my feelings."

And my heart broke because I can see the wolves mercilessly attacking my little lamb and knowing this will only escalate. I could send him on a separate van but how much do you isolate and point out differences? So for now, we are off to school at 7:10. We let Stefanie off first. It is about ten blocks to Chad's school. We take the same route every day. Even if Stefanie is ill and not going to school, we take the route past her school. We have the same conversation every morning after she gets out. "Will I get deaf just from hearing the loud noises of the kids in the gym? Does God know that will scare me and because He knows that will scare me He won't let that happen?" "Yes, Chad, God knows that would scare you and He won't let that happen. You can't go deaf from children's voices. God didn't make you to go deaf from people noises. It is only things like going up to a big jet engine and listening to noises like that."

"I won't get blind or lose my voice either?" "No, Chad, you won't get blind or lose your voice either." "And you won't get deaf or blind or lose your voice either?" "No, Chad, I can see and hear just fine and you can hear I haven't lost my voice."

"Good and you're still picking me up?" "Yes, Chad I am still picking you up. I will never forget you and leave you at school."

Or, if he is riding the bus home: "Nothing bad will happen on the bus will it? He won't forget to stop or change the route and you'll be waiting at the end of the walk?"

"Yes, Chad, Jim always remembers to stop, even when you and Stefanie don't ride, and he can't change the route because that would scare children and Mama's and Daddy's, and yes, I will be waiting at the end of the walk."

"Nothing bad will happen to me at school today? Nothing will take too long? Nothing will take forever?

"No, Chad, nothing will take too long. Nothing will take forever." Once again I can't promise nothing bad will happen.

By now we are at school. I tell him how much I love him, how proud of him I am. Until recently I only prayed silently this prayer: "God, I commit my angel to you. I can't protect him. I wish I could. But I can't. You made him this way so you have to take care of him. May the peace that passes all understanding keep his heart and mind in Christ Jesus. And someday would you give him a friend?"

Just recently, I have started to touch him and pray the blessing aloud. It may comfort him.

I don't just leave him to go in alone. I go with him. We did it that way the first day. So we do it every day. Up we go fifty seven steps.

I walk him inside, assure him that I will be there or waiting at the bus stop. Up he goes to face the wolves. All fourth and fifth graders at this school gather in the gym for the first ten minutes of school for announcements and chaos. This was too much for Chad. Noise, confusion, children hitting each other with backpacks. Snide comments about his value as he walked by. Perhaps kids not wanting to sit by him. I can't bear to hear it all. I chose a battle. Now he goes quietly up to his locker and puts his things away. Then into the quiet room of either the speech therapist, located next to his classroom, or his Special Education Manager, both gentle and loving ladies, and prepares for his day.

I go back home to get Matthew off to school.

I parent differently than I had planned. Because I don't want the disparity of treatment of the kids to be greater than I have to, I haven't placed the expectations on Matt and Stefanie that I had planned. Because I want them to grow up loving and not resenting their brother. Because I don't want to always hear "But Chad doesn't have to..." So most mornings I take Matt to school as well.

Then off to work. Today I am working on a big summer program for young adults ages 14-21. The first big event is a Summer Youth Job Fair which will be held in three weeks. We are frantically getting a mailing out to employers who may wish to do their summer hiring at the Fair. I work non-stop from the moment I walk in the door until I dash out the door at 1:45 to pick up the kids. Normally Stefanie and Chad ride the bus on Wed. and Thursday. But today is not a normal day for Chad. He is on a field trip to the area Inventor's Congress. Winners from various schools have their displays at Crossroad Mall.

(Chad did his project in January. He was supposed to work on it every-day over Christmas vacation but I said "Phooey". His invention was a Glow-In-The-Dark-Upper-Bunk-Holder for his water, tissues, and a luminous clock. He didn't win. But he did get his project done. And he uses it every night.)

Most kids look forward to field trips. Stefanie has one today, too. Her class is going skating at the National Hockey Arena at St. Cloud State University. She went to bed early last night to be sure she wouldn't get sick and miss out. She wears a special sweatshirt from Auntie Darlene with figure skaters and her skating necklace, also from Auntie Darlene, and digs our her skates and puts them in her special skating bag from guess who, and knows who she wants to sit with on the bus and can't wait.

Not so with Chad. And to top it off, a substitute teacher is on the agenda for the day.

Last night I said to Chad, "Chad tomorrow is Thursday. That's a day to take the bus. Will that work for you? And Mama will pick you up on Friday and we'll party until the cows come home."

"I guess so," he says reluctantly, which really means it isn't okay.

"Is there a problem? Tell me what you need, Chad."

"Well, it would make my field trip better if you picked me up.... (Pause)...And I have a substitute teacher tomorrow."

"That sounds like a lot of changes. I'd be happy to pick you up tomorrow. And that really was adult of you to tell Mama what you needed. I'm really proud of you."

So I pick up the kids. Steffy is just full of rap about her day and chats incessantly. I listen with half an ear. There is not a lot of time between the time her school lets out and Chad's and I don't want to be late for Chad. I was once. He was standing by the door, terrified. I could see his heart pounding through his shirt like a frightened bird. I felt like a monster. I assured him I would always come and told him what to do if he had to wait. But still I do everything in my power to move heaven and earth not to make him wait.

I dash up the stairs and am in time. He comes out. I ask him how his day was, and he volunteers information. He saw one neat exhibit: A Fish Alert. It was cool. And the substitute, Mr. Webster was really nice. Two bits of information volunteered which is amazing. Usually he will answer one question about his day and say, "I don't want to talk about it anymore." I don't press beyond that.

He is starving when he gets home. I have promised to take him for pizza after school as he has a freebie for reading a set number of books. I build in rewards of some kind almost every day so he has something to look forward to when he makes it through his day. His biggest reward, though, is just to be able to retreat to the comfort of his home. He grabs a bag of chips and something to drink and sits in the big chair in the living room, content and safe.

Mel has coffee made. Pours mine with cream; actually half and half. I used to drink it black but it is my concession to living life on the edge! My sister, Meg, set the example. When she turned forty she said, "Now if I want to have two cups of coffee a week, I will!" Obviously I come from a line of wild and crazy women.

There is apple pie to go with coffee. Mom was there the day before. Mel adds ice cream and serves. We have twenty five minutes before he goes to work. Stefanie won't leave us alone, but Chad is content to discharge in solitude.

He is looking forward to going to Coborn's, the grocery store, for new sugared drinks he saw a commercial on TV the night before. I told him to make a list and we would go to the store tomorrow. He used to be inconsolable if he thought of something he needed. Most often I ended up getting it. Not anymore. He can wait now. He has five things on his list, including the new sugared drinks. Despite the nutritional content, I will buy them just to get some food in his little body. I tell him after pizza we have two errands: Coborn's and Target. He is okay with that.

When Mel leaves for work at 3:00, we go for pizza. As I watch Stefanie color, I remember she had a couple of sore fingers a week or so before. I ask to see them. The tips of all fingers on her right hand are sore, skin wearing off. I see some signs on her right hand. Something is not right. I feel sick. We will go right home and call the doctor, I decide. They take their time eating. Then we go back home. Chad wants to go to Coborn's. I tell him we will after I speak with the doctor and it will just give the people at Coborn's more time to get the new drinks on the shelf. He is placated.

In time I speak with the nurse. She has no idea, either, and thinks it odd. She tells me to have Stefanie at Urgent Care in one hour. There is not time for both Coborn's and Target. Stefanie's teacher has gotten pop beads, of all things, there the day before. Steffy is dying for some. She is the one having the doctor appointment. I decide we go to Target first. I tell Chad we will go to Coborn's after the doctor. He asks how long it will be. I say, "It shouldn't take that long." We can't find the pop beads at Target. There are two Target stores in town. It has to be the other one. Steffy is very unhappy about it and tries to extract the promise we will go to the other Target right after the doctor and before Coborn's. I tell her we'll see.

We go to the Doctor.

Chad asks how long it will be until we get to Coborn's. And will it be closed when we get there. I tell him I think when the Doctor sees Stefanie's fingers he will know what to do and we won't have long to wait. And Coborn's won't be closed.

Chad paces around the lobby. He finds building blocks to play with but a toddler keeps coming over and knocking down his towers. He is frustrated. I tell him toddlers do that. He paces. Stefanie reads. I call Matthew. He is at Scott's and is wondering where we are. I tell him. He will go directly from Scott's to his Driver's Training class and we can pick him up at 8:50. Finally we get in the examining room. I take paper and pens out of my briefcase and they draw. Soon the doctor comes in. But he does not know what is going on with Stefanie's fingers. He calls in a pediatrician who has not gone home. They ask a lot of questions. Then consult outside. I hear low voices. He comes back in. They want to do some blood tests. And an x-ray and will see us after those are done. He tells me they want to rule out some more serious problems. I sense concern. Chad has finished his picture--a twelve pound northern. He is getting fidgety. He asks again when we will be going to Coborn's and will it have closed before we get there. I explain again it is open all night.

We go down to the lab. Buoyed by the promise that I will go to the other Target for the pop beads, Stefanie doesn't make a fuss. But she doesn't know she is getting blood taken out of her arm. That hasn't happened before. I decide not to explain it in advance. We wait a few minutes. Chad has reached his limit. Tears are in his eyes. He pleads for us to go to Coborn's and then home. I need to go home, he says. I tell him we have to do several things for Stefanie first to be sure she is okay. He asks how long it will be. I say, I hope not too long. But I know it could be. The lab tech comes and explains and Stefanie asks me to hold her fist while it is done. Chad doesn't want to remain in the lobby but he doesn't belong back by Stefanie. I am needed with Stefanie and with Chad. But I can't be both places. I go with Stefanie. But I stand so Chad can see me. He has tears in his eyes. So does Stefanie. It is scary. And it is hurting. And she is getting sick. The test is done. I take her back to the lobby. She is ready to faint. Chad is trying to keep the tears from flowing. That embarrasses him. He pleads with me to go. I put Stefanie's head between her legs. It doesn't help. She is feeling terrible. Chad asks how soon can we go and will Coborn's still be open and will they for sure have what we need and can we go right home afterwards because he needs to go home. And sick as she is Stefanie hears it and moans "I'm sick and I have to have my pop beads."

I carry her into a room off the lab that has a table and put her on it. Chad follows, pleading to go home and trying to keep from crying. I stabilize Stefanie, and get a cold rag for her head. The X-ray tech comes for Stefanie. I tell her she will have to wait. Chad paces. His neck is blotching and his cheeks are starting to get too pink. It is not hot in the room. I am feeling dizzy. I suspect it my blood pressure going up. I don't know how to handle Stefanie and Chad at the same time. I sense I am pushing Chad farther than he can be pushed but I don't know what to do. I keep reassuring him and Stefanie. Chad pleads to go home after Coborn's. Stefanie is feeling better. She is adamant on the pop beads.

Stefanie has her x-ray. We go back to the Urgent Care Lobby to wait. Stefanie wants to be held. So does Chad. There are people in the lobby. Chad doesn't want anyone to see him cry. So he holds it in. And his neck gets more blotched and his cheeks look like he has frost-bite. He gets up and kicks a toy truck across the room and into the wall several times, makes a couple of towers with the building blocks, plays momentarily with my matchbook calculator. He is beyond amusement. Stefanie is now coloring. I hold Chad. He keeps begging to go. I think he would even give up Coborn's if it meant he could go home. I have pushed him farther than I have ever seen him pushed. I am still dizzy. Things are spinning for me when I get up. I know it is the stress. I am worried about Chad. I take out my ace in the hole - my cell phone in my briefcase. Even that does not interest Chad. We suffer in the lobby for half an hour.

Finally we are called back in the room. The doctor says the prelimi-nary tests have ruled out Kawasaki's disease. I ask what it is. All I hear is that it causes serious problems with the heart. I feel like I could puke. Chad is beside himself. Tears. Hands thru his hair. Twisting. Turning. Blotching. Pinching his neck and cheeks. Close to a panic. If he notices, the doctor says nothing. We get a prescription and some instructions. And head to the pharmacy.

It takes ten minutes. Chad is beyond himself. I hold him when he lets me and assure him we will go to Coborn's. He begs to go home afterward. Stefanie insists on the pop beads for her suffering. "I am

43

the one getting the blood taken Chad. I'm the one who fainted. I get the pop beads." Chad begs to have the upstairs TV when we get home to watch *Cats Don't Dance*. (The downstairs VCR is not working so they have to take turns.)

We make it to the car. I wonder if I can drive. I am so dizzy. We make it to Coborn's. Forget buying groceries. We buy only what is on Chad's list, and decaf coffee, and a couple items Stefanie wants. Chad does okay. He thinks we are going home. When it is apparent we are heading to Target, he gets hysterical. He asks if he gets the upstairs TV to watch *Cats Don't Dance*. Stefanie assures him he can have the upstairs TV because she will be working on her pop beads. We make it to Target. It is 7:30. Chad is worried that we won't be home until after 8 and he won't have time to finish *Cats Don't Dance* before bedtime at 9:20. And Stefanie is insisting that she gets to watch her WEE Sing movie before bed, but will let Chad watch his first.

The pop beads are not at this Target. We are goal orientated. We ask every possible person who could know. Stefanie insists we check every part of the store. I tell her we are leaving. Now.

As we leave the store she announces that since she doesn't have pop beads, she is no longer okay with Chad having the upstairs VCR to watch *Cats Don't Dance*. We are at the car. I put Chad in the front; Stefanie is in the back. Chad freaks. Stef persists. I tell her that we have pushed Chad too far and to back off. She doesn't. Chad freaks more. I am trying to drive. I am spinning and am just trying to make it the four miles home. I wonder if the kids would think of taking out my cell phone to call for help if I pass out. I order her to be quiet. She begins crying. Chad settles down. Tears well up in my eyes and fall all the way home. The car is silent except for muffled sobs from the back seat and the ironically mellow sounds of Christian radio.

We pull into the garage. Both kids scatter. Chad immediately takes his stash of goodies into the living room and puts on *Cats Don't Dance*.

I find Stefanie in my bed, sobbing.

"Mind if I cry with you?" I ask. I take off her glasses and mine. I crawl under the comforter beside her. She rolls over into my arms and we both bawl. Hard. And we talk. Perhaps the best talk we have ever had.

She tells me it's too hard for her and that Chad always gets his way but she needs things for her life, too, and doesn't get them. She spills her guts. I listen. I tell her I'm sorry her life is so hard. I remind her that Chad is autistic. And she says, I'm autistic, too, And I say, no, Stefanie, you aren't autistic. You have needs but you aren't autistic. And she cries more. And I cry. And I tell her what it is like for Chad. How people look at him weird. And tease him. And how he can't make friends. And that he will always be like that until heaven and how it won't ever change and how hard his life will be. And how hard her life is because of it. And I tell her I know I make mistakes sometimes and make the wrong choice of whose needs are most important because hers are just as important as Chad's. And I ask her to forgive me.

"Can't God change him and make him better?" she asks.

"Yes."

"So if we pray God will change him?"

"No, probably not."

"Why not?"

"Because God usually doesn't' change a person once He makes him autistic.

"Why? Doesn't God know how hard it is?" "Doesn't God see you cry, Mama?"

I suspect I have never had a more difficult theological question raised.

"Yes, God knows. God sees Mama cry. But God has reasons we can't

45

understand, Stefanie. I don't understand everything but I know God's plans are good and right. And His plan is for Chad to be autistic. And His plan for Stefanie is to have an autistic brother. And His plan for Mama is to have an autistic son."

And I sob holding my little red haired angel, thinking of how much it was like the conversation I had with Chad when I told him he was autistic. Sobbing because I can't change things and make everything right.

I go on and tell her what it's like to be the mama and have Matt and Chad and her all needing things and many times I can't do what all three need and I don't know what to do. And that I know it is terribly hard for her. But Chad has no one to make his world safe but us and what does she think we should do?

And she says "We have to take care of Chad." And she strokes my face and holds me and then leaves to go to the living room to join Chad and they watch *Cats Don't Dance*.

I lie for a few minutes, too dizzy and spinning to move, but it's 8:15. Matt has to be picked up at 8:50. And there are lunches to be packed, clothes to be taken out and ironed for tomorrow, homework, showers....

Chad has calmed down. I start the work. We pick up Matt. Since they can't be left alone, they have to come with. Steffy hits the shower and starts her homework at 9:15. After homework is done, Mama's help is needed, she turns on the movie she wanted and watches fifteen minutes. She crawls into bed at 10:00. Bedtime is 8:30.

Chad, who has a self-determined bedtime of 9:20, is late. He doesn't get in the shower til 9:24. He is worried about getting late to bed. I assure him he will be okay and I will wake him up 15 minutes later in the morning. That won't work he tells me as he has to see the opening of Timon and Pumbaa. So we agree on a 6:15 wake up and I'll tickle his nose and carry him to the sofa so he is sure to wake up. I assure him I will pick him up after school tomorrow and we'll party till the cows come home.

10:00. The two littlest are in bed. Matt has done real well on his practice driving test final. We go through the fifty questions. I do terrible and admit that if I had to take the test I would flunk. Wait. He also had a quiz tonight he did real well on. We look at that as well. And he tells me some of the cool things he has learned. And we chat about that. We talk about his Spanish test. And does he need to go to Scott's in the morning. And is there anything he needs to do in any of his classes before the quarter ends tomorrow? And I check more thoroughly the gash on his nose from where a locker smacked his face and we determine his nose is not broken and we won't have to head to the Emergency room.

I am too tired to shower or iron. I am starving but too tired to chew. I realize I have not eaten since the apple pie. Matt kisses me goodnight and is off to bed. I go in the bathroom, wash my face and slip into my gown. And stumble into my dark bedroom not bothering to so much as turn on the light. In the pitch blackness I don't see the body lying under the covers warming my side of the bed. I feel only a soft kiss on my cheek as Matt slips out the other side and goes to his room. My eyes once again fill with tears for the sweet and tender mercy of my beloved fifteen year old son. Spent, I fall asleep.

Tomorrow is another day.

(Note to reader: One friend told me he was so exhausted after reading this chapter he needed a nap. If you need to stop reading and make a pot of coffee, I totally understand.)

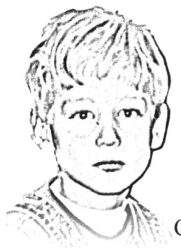

Chapter 9

# *"I Keep Dreaming of Things to Get Easier"*

"Mom," lamented Chad one day upon arriving home from another taxing day at school, "I keep dreaming of things to get easier."

Frankly, Chad, so do I!

Chad is now fifteen and while we've learned a lot about living with and even embracing autism, it doesn't get easier. The most heart-breaking experience as a mother is to observe his isolation and be powerless to make right the things in his world.

He knows he's autistic and is able to express this at appropriate times.
> "I can't help it; I'm autistic."
> "This is the worst autism I've had."

He knows he's God's special missionary, God's special agent-James

Bond so-to-speak. He has a strong sense of mission and purpose in life because of this.

> "There's nothing I'd rather be than Jesus' missionary. And there's no exception to that."

At times he gets discouraged.

> "Doesn't Jesus know His boy needs to be with him?"
> "I have feelings just like normal people."

And once, "I forgive Jesus" (for making me autistic). Such honesty!

Fear is a constant companion of the autistic.

> "The thing I was most worried about today was going back to school. The thing I was most excited about today was going back home after school."

> "I'm scared of school. I like to be with my brother."

Loneliness is another companion. He has never made a true friend. The most heartbreaking experience I ever witnessed was when he almost made a friend. He was in fifth grade. The boy agreed to come over for a play date and then canceled. Chad was devastated. "It feels like my heart has broken in a million pieces." Another date was set and again canceled. Unwilling to be hurt like that again, Chad never has put his heart back on front street. It was after this experience that his obsessive compulsive behaviors started and our foray into the maze of counseling and prescription meds began. The precipitating cause was shockingly clear. And he has never recovered.

> "Don't you know how it feels to be left out?"
> "If I can't play with them, can I just be with them and watch?"

> Dogs make excelent pets.
> Dogs are good company.
> Dogs can do tricks like playing catch.
> Dogs like to go on walks and get exercize.
> Dogs will like you even when other people don't.
> Age 11

I think of how many times the best players are sidelined during the exhibition season, but how do I explain that to Chad?

I am told by school personnel that his peers are supportive and protective and I am thankful. I know, however, that's not always the case. One day two fellow students turned the bathroom lights off when Chad was still there. Just to torment. Chad was terrified. The principal tracked down the culprits and made them apologize.

> Dear Chad,
> I'm sorry for turning the lights out on you and I hope we can still be friends. I am VREY VREY Sorry.
> From T.W.

> Dear Chad,
> I am sorry for scaring you yesterday in the bathroom by flicking the light off and on. I didn't mean to scare you. I didn't know you would be scared and scream. Please forgive me. I am very sorry.
> Sincerely,
> E.W.

One hopes they truly meant it.

Chad is now in high school. I can only imagine what comes his way. While he says it is going well, I observed him one morning waiting for class to begin. His hands just shook. I sobbed all the way to my office. And his father observed him getting shoved into a locker, calling on all of his personal control not to go beat up the bully then and there.

I love his creativity. He had an idea for a game at the fair based on a dream: Dig-For-A-Dog. You'd hide a bunch of puppies under something with spots marked. People could pay money and dig in a spot and if they found a puppy, they could keep it! Sure beats the other stupid ways you throw away your money at the fair!

He was in a play once in third grade. He was the third farmhand in "The Boy Who Cried Wolf". He had two lines which he can recite with pride to this day.

"Look it's the shepherd boy. The one folks are talking about."

"We don't believe you."
Talk about being relegated to the most humble acting role. Interesting that the line spoke of a shepherd boy! I think of the words from a song which remind me so much of Chad: "Where others see a shepherd boy, God may see a king…." [4] Chad has taught me we need to re-define greatness.

Inspired by his acting role, he wrote a play, his rendition of "How the Tortoise Beat the Hare" which he and Stefanie performed at the Nelson Christmas, my family's yuletide gathering.

There's moments when he's so "normal" I laugh.

This note left for me in bold letters one day:

MOM
I RAN AWAY.
CHAD

And this sweet note left for me on my birthday.

Mom,
I love you in all my heart. I wish you happy birthday from me to you. I love you no matter what comes between us.
Yours truely
Chad

He says so many wonderful things. Here is a sampler for you to enjoy. "Well, it certainly wasn't the best day of my life!"(First day of school in sixth grade)

"I sure hope we don't get locked out of our room when we're naked. It'd be so embarrassing. And cold too."
(Staying overnight in a motel)

"I really need to pull myself together."

"I don't think I've ever been quite this happy." (On the way to Gull Lake for our family Memorial Day weekend tradition.) Of course there's the other side. The side I see more often. Truly no parent has answers for questions that their kids ask. But many times they are predictable like "What holds up the air?" I get this kind: "Can my middle finger turn into a piccolo?" or "Can anyone swallow Canada?"

When he was thirteen he wrote a collection of stories. Some new; some twists on old stories or stories he'd just read. Enjoy some of the titles and descriptions in his words and spelling:

- Wallace and Gromit and the Lost Piggy Bank
- Christmas G'Night
    You'll G'laugh!
    You'll G'cry!
    You'll G'howl!

    Merry G'Christmas to you all too. Then they all looked at their presents. Just what I always wanted, said Sam, a g'pink tux. Oh, said Sandi, a fancy g'piggy bank. All right, said Seth, a "gwoppy cushion….Hey Wow, said Grandpapa, g'blue under-pance. Ooh, said Grandmama, g'laxitive. Well it was quite a fun Christmas g'night….

- My Favorite Clocks
- The Missing Necklace
    A Folks Tale for All Ages
- The Autistic Rhino
    Sarah is an autistic rhino that works for the king. The king's name is William E. Lawrence but everyone calls him King William. Anyway King William knows that Sarah is autistic, so he tries to go as easy on Sarah as possible. …Sarah did anything for King William. She helped him put on his night-cap, she helped him put on his slippers, she cooked for him, she tucked him in at bedtime. King William liked Sarah very much. In fact he never wanted her to leave his kingdom cause he thought Sarah was the sweetest rhino that God ever made. Whenever King William had parties, Sarah would cook for

him and his guests….And whenever King William got thirsty, Sarah would give him an unalcoholic martini. Sarah was such a nice and autistic rhino indeed.

- The Happy King Samuel

   A long time ago….there lived a happy king named Samuel. Anyway Samuel was different than the other kings. You see, King Samuel would take his violin and sing Oh I Dreamed I Was in Paradise every Monday. Well the problem was King Samuel had three royal servents named Edmund, Harry and Rayburn. And they were sick of him being so happy.

   "Good afternoon, Sire!" smiled Edmund, "I think you need a bath." "A bath?" smiled King Samuel, "I don't smell too bad, do I? Besides I've taken a bath two days ago." "I know, Sire," said Edmund, "But you should take one just in case."

   Well that's almost the end of our story I just have one thing to tell you. Edmund, Harry and Rayburn loved Samuel's song of Paradise, They became just as happy as him. Each day on their break they'd sing and dance. But there was one problem. King Samuel got sick of them being so happy each day so he tried to think up a nasty sceam to stop them from being so happy. The End.

- The Green Café
- Wallace and Gromit and the Great West

My favorite is his rendition of Daniel in the Lion's Den.

   (After Daniel was able to tell King Darius what the king had dreamed) The king was outrageously pleased….He asked Daniel if he would like to be second in command. Daniel said, "Yes!" Wow! Daniel had never been so happy in his life. He even thanked God for making him so wise and everything going good for a few days."

   (When King Darius implemented the law that his people could only pray to him) Well the wise men spread the new law all over Babylon. And everyone in Babylon heard the new law especially Daniel, but when Daniel heard about the new law he ran home and started praying to god. He thanked him for everything good in life and he even thanked god for giving him the courage to do what's right even though it could get him in trouble.

(Upon being thrown into the lions' den) First it was quiet in the lion's den. Daniel wasn't scared at first. But then there was growling. How unpleasant. It was no picnic for poor Daniel.

He saw the lions and got a bit scared but at that moment Daniel saw a bright and beautiful light. The lions paused. It was an angel. The angel sat next to Daniel. The lions stopped growling. The lions began to like Daniel and didn't want to hurt him. Daniel went to the lions and patted them. The next morning King Darius ran to the lions to see if Daniel was alive. Because the king loved Daniel and didn't want him to get hurt. "Daniel," cried King Darius, "Are you still alive?" "Hello, sire!" said Daniel. "I gotta say goodbye to my friends." Daniel said goodbye to the lions and climbed back up and King Darius was happy for Daniel and made a new law for everyone in Babylon to only pray to Daniel's God.

Chad's most striking attribute is his love for God and his concern that no one spends eternity in hell. He can't bear to think of anyone being there.
> "Can God minister to people in hell if they don't get breakfast?"

His heart is focused on the eternal.
> "Jesus really saved me and I'm forever grateful."
> "Sometimes I stare at the sky and think about Jesus and heaven. Whenever I see a sunset I think about Jesus and heaven."

This was his response to a question asked on a school assignment:
> If I could do anything I wanted, I would…
> "I would like to worship Jesus."

Well meaning acquaintances/friends give me books and articles on

55

the latest treatments and cures for autism obviously with the intent that I change him from autistic to "normal" or some semblance thereof.

My heart rebels. Why? Why would I wish to change a pure and innocent and undivided heart for God into someone who is more capable of contributing to the Gross National Product of a global society? Why must he be the smartest (in the eyes of academia), most talented child as defined by society? The world has everything backwards. People should be asking ME how to change their brilliant, talented child into a child with Chad's attributes, values and priorities. That's what SHOULD be happening. How can we be so blind that we do not recognize treasure when it's right in front of our eyes?

My son is wonderful, talented, and beautiful; entrusted by Almighty God with a special mission; living *THE* purpose driven life. Chad is a strong and courageous warrior, a brave and experienced soldier and fighter, God's mighty warrior on an incredible assignment.

May 2, 1999 (age 12)
The Nelsons stand holding hands at the foot of the walking bridge, at the Rum River in Milaca. We've driven from the Baptist Church where we'd all gathered for Sunday morning worship and communion.

The previous fall Chad had come to me with a request. "Mom, I want to get baptized as soon as Uncle Tim can come home and do it. I love Jesus so much. I want him to know that so I want to get baptized."

The sun shines warmly on the assembled group: Grandma Nelson, aunts, uncles, cousins, brother, sister, mom and dad. Daddy, Uncle Roger, Grandma Nelson and Uncle Tim pray blessings upon Chad: prayers for God's Spirit to be on Chad's life in a special way, prayers of thankfulness.

"You have given our family a gift we don't deserve, but we accept him this special gift." Eyes that see Chad's true value, waterlogged with tears.

A little hand in the big hand of the uncle he was named for, Chad and Uncle Tim step gingerly into the cold, waist high waters. Daddy gives Tim a hanky. Theoretically to put over Chad's nose. Tim explains again to Chad what he will do. He asks Chad for a profession of faith and Chad enthusiastically complies.

Tim takes a baggie with an index card out of his pocket.

> Chad, you are God's warrior. May God's Word be in your heart like a burning fire, shut up in your bones, may you not be able to hold it back. Have no fear on any side. For the Lord is with thee as a mighty warrior. Therefore those who attack you will stumble and not prevail. They will be greatly ashamed, for you, Chad Timothy, were born a warrior of God, to love God and to fight valiantly for His Kingdom.

> *"I have bestowed strength on a warrior: I have exalted a young man from among the people."* (Psalm 89:19 NIV)

The blessing concluded, Tim's strong arms gently lower Chad into the frigid waters.

> "I baptize you in the name of the Father, the Son, and the Holy Spirit."

They come out of the waters, Tim's arm still lovingly around Chad. "Are you proud of me, Mama", chattering teeth notwithstanding Chad says to me. "Are you proud of me, Mama? I'm proud of myself. I love Jesus so much."

We hurry him to the car to change. And we're off to Hardees for lunch. We have much to celebrate.

Warriors are a breed set apart. Many are soldiers; few are warriors.

It's okay to dream of things to get easier, Chad. I do, too. And someday they will. I promise. But until then, God's mighty warrior, be brave and strong. God is with you until the battle is won.

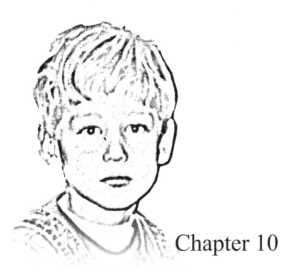

# Chapter 10

# *Musings on Chad's 21ST Birthday*

It's a cold January afternoon. Snow showers are falling outside the coffee shop window. A piping hot cup of hazelnut, with cream, is my only table companion.

It's Chad's twenty first birthday—his golden birthday. It's a school holiday and he's at home in his room listening to a new C/D—John Denver's Greatest Hits. Matt has the day off from college, and is watching fishing shows in the living room with his dad. Stefanie just drove off in her little Corolla to begin her second semester of college.

Twenty one years ago, God's special agent, Chad Timothy, entered this world on special assignment. How fitting that he should become a James Bond walking encyclopedia virtually impossible to stump!

As the snow descends, so do my tears. Tears of exhaustion, grief, joy, thankfulness, and hope. Absolute certainty that eternity will make right everything in this topsy-turvy world of mine.

This past Christmas, I went to a concert at my secretary, Allison's, church. The preschoolers marched by, singing their little hearts out. I remember being that young, singing my little heart out, loving Jesus with all my heart. How could I have known the challenges and pain the next fifty years would hold? That it would be such an exhausting, solitary and perilous journey?

My world looks nothing like I thought it would. My parenting, my marriage did not turn out as I expected. The war for my heart rages— with some victories and some stunning defeats. I am weary in body and spirit.

The snow is intensifying outside the window. I get myself another cup of hazelnut and pray for Stefanie's safety as she travels the three hours back to college through the snow. What a pure joy is my red haired daughter and how I treasure Matt, my beloved first born Gift of God.

And I affirm with everything in me that Chad is a gift of God, a joy, a privilege, an unspeakable treasure. He has embraced his life purpose of loving God. To know him is to love him and to marvel at his courage and love for God.

This past year, my Mom died. We sent her into eternity as a family, providing hospice, digging the grave, making the vault, doing everything in the memorial service. The church was packed for the memorial service, a rainbow of sizes and backgrounds and personalities, all with one common denominator: our sweet Mama Delight.

As the last notes of the prelude fell from Stefanie's flute, a handsome young man in black slacks, a black and white striped dress shirt and black silk tie walked up the steps to the podium to give the call to worship. And in a strong voice, Chad read the verses we had selected to honor his beloved grandma.

This morning, on his twenty first birthday, I asked him, "If you could have chosen to be autistic or not autistic, which would you have chosen?" He replied immediately but thoughtfully, "I'd have been autistic. I accept how God made me. I'm glad it's not Matt or Stefanie. The Lord will be proud of me because of how I handled autism. And, Mom, I'll know the things I don't know here."

Living with Chad is like living with Jesus.

No mother could ask for a greater treasure.

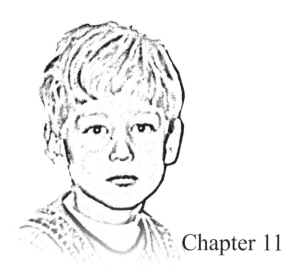

## Chapter 11

# *Braveheart, Chad Style*

You are requested to be the guest speaker at the annual fundraiser of a non-profit organization serving individuals with disabilities. It is being held at the most elegant conference center in the community. It is expected that over two hundred community members will be in attendance. A silent auction is being held and a formal dance will follow the gourmet dinner and your speech. Dress is formal. You will be seated at the head table with the mayor who will be introducing you.

I believe I am hearing an immediate and resounding "Absolutely not! You couldn't pay me to do that!"

If you are like the majority of Americans, fear of public speaking is your worst fear. Beating out fear of death and prancing in public sans garments.

Let's compound the situation and make this request of an autistic individual who experiences additional challenges with communication and social interaction. A recipe for disaster. Or remarkable bravery.

This very request was made of Chad by the Executive Director of one of the agencies providing his day services. And his response was "yes".

As with any keynote speaker, it was left to Chad to write his speech. Other than a few prompts regarding topics that might be of interest to his listeners, the entire speech is pure Chad.

On the night of the annual fundraiser, after a family prayer for God's peace and power to rest upon Chad, his father and I proudly escorted the keynote speaker to the conference center. Later Chad told me "I was more confident than afraid. I felt quite certain that I could do it and I could pull it off."

When the mayor shared that the guest speaker was an individual receiving services from the agency, a hush descended on the crowd and a handsome young man dressed in black headed to the podium.

You could have heard a pin drop as he read his thoughtfully composed words:

*Good Evening.*

*My name is Chad Brenden and I'm a 22 year old missionary with autism who has been coming to Opportunity Manor since October of 2008. I call myself a missionary because my family and I are devoted Christians.*

*I come to Opportunity Manor four days a week and I'm in the Pathways to Opportunities Program.*

*On Monday, I work in the cantina, do inventory for the cantina, and sometimes I do internet research.*

*On Tuesday, I am with a cooking class and do recreational activities.*

*I have learned how to cook things like grilled cheese, cookies and enchiladas. My favorite thing I've made is spaghetti. Sometimes I bring the recipes home and make them there. Cooking is fun.*

*On Wednesday, I volunteer at the St. Cloud Hospital in Riverfront Dining. Some of the tasks I do there include: organizing silverware, cleaning tables, organizing food like chips, salad dressings, candy and milks. I enjoy my hospital volunteering a lot. I like helping people.*

*Thursday is my favorite day of the week. I am with a Thursday fieldtrip group. A group of us go to fun and educational places in the community. Some of the places we have gone include: Bernicks Pepsi, Best Buy, the Sauk Rapids Fire Station, Viking Coke, and Coborns Superstore.*

*Once a month we get to go bowling. I have gotten a strike or 2 on occasion.*

*I have learned important new skills being in the Pathways Program. When I came here, I had a fear of getting chemicals on my hands. I have conquered that fear and I am quite proud of that.*

*The people who work with me here are kind and respectful.*

*My hobbies include: watching movies, listening to music, reading the Bible and writing James Bond Trivia cards.*

*I have been James Bond savvy for 7 years. I have all his movies and I have written 909 trivia cards. Most of them have 2 questions. I'm pretty hard to stump!*

*An example of a James Bond trivia question is: So far how many James Bond movies are there?*

*The answer is 25. That was pretty easy.*

*Here's a stumper:*
*On Goldfinger when Auric Goldfinger showed up in the plane*

*James Bond said to Auric Goldfinger "Way to go on the promotion Goldfinger. Are you having dinner at the White House too?" What does Mr. Goldfinger say to James Bond as he points his golden gun at him?*

*The answer is: "In 2 hours I shall be in Cuba and you have interfered with my plans for the last time Mr. Bond."*

*Did anyone get those answers?*

*I always thought autism was one of the main keys to becoming James Bond savvy.*

*I'm pretty excited for my future. I don't know what my plans are exactly. I would like to stay in this community.*

*Thank you for coming this evening and supporting Opportunity Manor.*

The mesmerized crowd broke into instantaneous applause. The mayor, who had been standing off to the side beaming as Chad read, walked to the podium, shaking Chad's hand and thanking him.

The James Bond trivia questions had elicited quite the response from the guests! Among the guests was a gentleman who had just been in the news for winning big on the TV program, Jeopardy.

The mayor had Chad pose two trivia questions to the Jeopardy winner, neither of which was answered correctly. Which had the mayor, Jeopardy winner, audience – and Chad – laughing. What a delightful moment, everyone drawn into the charm of the Special Agent with autism.

After graciously fielding the thanks of numerous guests, the guest speaker made his way out of the conference center and to the safe refuge of his home. All the stress of speaking had caught up with him and his cheeks were flushed a beet red indicative of an anxiety attack.

As I tucked him into bed, telling him once again how proud of him I was, he said, "This was the bravest thing I have ever done! It was impossible but the Lord helped me."

Yes, Chad, it is the bravest thing you have ever done. It was the bravest thing anyone could have done. And yes, you and the Lord did the impossible.

And I added this amazing experience of God's Brave Warrior to the treasure box of my heart.

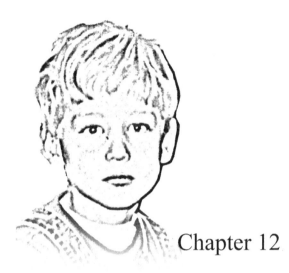

Chapter 12

# *Smiles in the Emergency Room*

It looked like an ordinary tick bite, but the story that goes along with it is far from ordinary.

We had just come home from a lunch date when Chad told me his leg itched. In checking I found a wood tick, attached to the back of his leg. It appeared to have been there for a couple of days, unnoticed by Chad until it began itching.

The area around it was already a little red. I removed the tick, applying home remedies.

The next morning, I checked and the area was swollen and red. A call was made to the doctor, and an appointment made. The doctor prescribed oral antibiotics and told me to keep an eye on it.

The next day, the area had continued to swell and looked very infected. We made a trip back to the doctor who this time ordered an injection of antibiotics. I made sure the doctor was aware of Chad's allergy to penicillin products. We were told to wait in the lobby for a certain amount of time to be sure there was no reaction to the injection as Chad had not received that medication before.

All was well. I called my husband who came and picked up Chad and I returned to work.

It was early afternoon and both my husband and Chad laid down for a nap. As Chad laid there he realized something was wrong and went into the bathroom to look in the mirror. Seeing his face red and swollen, he went into his father's bedroom and told him he felt funny.

One look at Chad, and my husband was on the phone to me and getting Chad into the car to rush to the ER less than five minutes away.

My office was only about three blocks from the hospital so I was running into the ER as they drove up.

Not only Chad's face was swelling, but also his body. He could hardly speak.

Would I lose my son?

Emergency personnel sprang into action to save his life.

I had not been told the name of the drug Chad had been given, so the staff desperately called the clinic to get the information. (I was told by hospital staff that this drug is not one that should be used with individuals with allergies to penicillin.)

Not surprisingly the major concern was to make sure his airway did not close. What seemed like forever was probably less than an hour, and Chad began to stabilize.

Due to the severity of the reaction and some complications, Chad was admitted to the hospital.

Later that evening when Chad was resting comfortably and we were alone, I told him once again how proud I was of him for being so brave.

"I was brave, wasn't I Mom?" was his reply, adding "I'm proud of myself, too. And God was proud of me."

I then asked him about something that had baffled me since he laid helpless on the gurney in the ER. "When I met you and Dad in the Emergency Room and all the time you were there with the doctors and nurses frantically working on you, you had a big smile. Your face was all puffy but you were smiling. Did you know you were smiling?"

Chad nodded in the affirmative so I proceeded to ask him why he was smiling.

I was not prepared for his response. "I was happy."

Not understanding, I asked in clarification, "You were smiling because you were happy?"

Chad nodded again.

I probed further. "Can you tell me why you were happy?"

Seriously and thoughtfully Chad shared, "You told me that God knows just the right time and the right way for me to die. I've been waiting my whole life for today to come."

Scarcely believing my ears, I said, "So you were smiling because you thought you were dying?"

He nodded and I turned my face to look out the window so he would not be frightened by my falling tears.

May it also be said of me when I am moments from death that I am smiling from ear to ear in trust and anticipation.

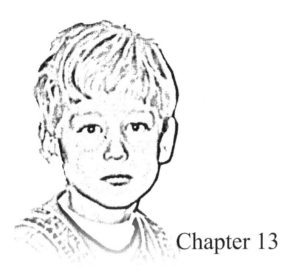

## Chapter 13

# *A Thank You Like None Other*

It was the most beautiful example of God's grace that I have ever seen. Not surprisingly it came from Chad.

Chad's vocational options are limited. At twenty six, we are all working with Chad to find a "fit".

In high school and his bridging program, Chad had opportunities to work alongside a school para-professional in a video store, public library, and school library.

Since Chad aged out of his bridging program at twenty one, he has been receiving services from two agencies which serve adults with disabilities. Presently, one primarily works with Chad on independent living skills, socialization, and provides a job coach to be with him so he can volunteer at the hospital in the laundry and dining room. The other assists with job coaching for Chad to be on a cleaning crew, where faithfully, hour after hour, he vacuums hallways and cleans windows and vents for Jesus.

When Chad was twenty three, the opportunity arose for him to have a paid internship. The site identified was one of the nicest restaurants in St. Cloud and Chad had the job of rolling silverware.

Three mornings a week, Chad would go to this restaurant. After washing his hands, he would get the napkins, silverware, and bucket for rolled silverware, and bring them to a table or booth in the rear of the restaurant. A job coach gave him initial instruction and popped in perhaps weekly to see how it was going. Chad's job was to roll the silverware in either paper or linen napkins and put them in the bucket to be used when the restaurant opened and service to customers began. Chad worked diligently on his tasks, occasionally stopping long enough to get a glass of pop graciously provided.

Chad's work habits are thorough, methodical, and slow.

His quality of work was excellent; speed problematic. Had he been with his present job coach, the dauntless Kristine Hollingsworth, I'm positive a way would have been found to help Chad increase his speed.

Chad loved the job. One of his favorite parts was making sure that every piece of silverware was clean before he rolled it. He told me that as he worked he often thought of "the dirty fork scene" from Monty Python's *And Now for Something Completely Different*.

Not being a Monty Python fan like my kids, I had to ask him to explain.

In Chad's words, Graham Chapman and his girlfriend were having dinner at a fancy five star restaurant. Graham says, "I've got a little bit of a dirty fork!" Restaurant employees become apologetic and try to remedy the situation and Graham tries not to make a big scene. However, it causes absolute chaos, including employees having meltdowns. When it ends, Graham looks into the camera and says with a little smile, "At least I didn't tell them about the dirty knife!"

The manager was very respectful and kind to Chad, but while Chad's attitude and winsomeness were exceptional, his speed was not. Less than four months later, Chad was told he the job would be ending.

Chad's reported that the job coach told him the reasons for letting him go were that " the restaurant was not in the position to be hiring anyone for this position and that the restaurant manager saw a lot more to me than just silverware rolling and thought it was time for me to move on to other jobs."

You and I know otherwise.

Chad's response was "I am a little bit sad about leaving because it was a cool job, but I am glad I lasted as long as I did."

On the last day, the manager was not there to say goodbye.

When he went to his office the next day, a thank you note in Chad's distinctive printing was waiting.

*(Name of Manager),*
*Thank you for all my months of working at (Name of Restaurant). I sure learned a lot and met a lot of great people.*
*Thank you. Chad*

Imagine getting a thank you note from a young man with a disability just "fired" from his job!

Grace! Pure, simple, unmerited, unequalled grace!

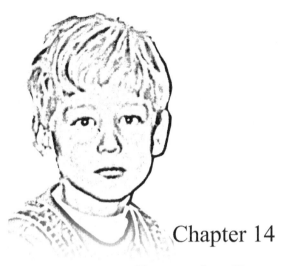

# Chapter 14

## *Cosmic Drama*

I had a very strange experience several years ago. In a conversation with a business colleague in our community, I threw out an idea for a musical. It happened that this colleague was also the owner and artistic director of a professional theatre in our city. Cutting to the chase, *Fishing Widows: The Reel Story* became one of the seven shows of the professional season several years later with my being the playwright and lyricist.

(Rest assured I am fully qualified to write a musical. My musical background consists of taking piano lessons from a backwoods teacher for one or two years when I was in early grade school. Putting on Christmas programs with about sixteen other country school cronies over a half century ago is the only experience on my theatrical performance résumé. Add to this, my training in writing comes only from the usual high school English classes and freshman English in college. How the show came to be can only be described as a God-thing which perhaps I will share at another time in another venue.)

In writing this show, I received the great gift of insight into God as the playwright of a cosmic drama and that my life is only understood from this perspective.

This Cosmic Drama from eternity past to eternity future, was planned in the mind and heart of God before the world began. My character was written into this drama, with absolute purpose and timing and a role which is essential to the full drama. I cannot understand the drama extracting only my small role with limited lines and interactions.

This is true of my life. This is true of Chad's life. This is true of your life. Each of our roles are essential to but cannot be understood apart from the entire drama.

We make this life larger than it is. The largeness of life is the Drama that the Playwright has written. Individual roles often do not make sense until you can look back from the vantage point of the end of the drama and see how each role was essential and how each conflict added to the powerful conclusion.

Chad and I walk in awe of being written into the script, giving our best Academy Award winning performances, awaiting with great anticipation Opening Night of the Cosmic Drama when we will see and know that the Drama would have been incomplete without our roles written just as they were.

And we will join in the Applause of Heaven over the Drama of Dramas which never ends.

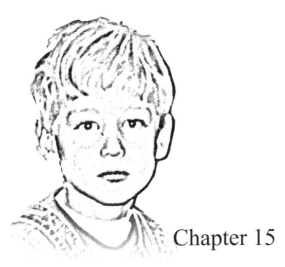

Chapter 15

# *Living Under the Mystery*

Embracing your role in the Cosmic Drama requires a life of living under the mystery.

I find it rather ironic how most people say they love mystery. Mystery novels, mystery movies – ask yourself, your friends, and see if that isn't true. Yet, when it comes to God, many of these same people say they want a god they can fully understand. There is no place for mystery when it comes to matter of faith.

I hate mystery books and movies. There is so much mystery in my life, why would I want to add more?

We can know only some things about God. It is not possible to understand many aspects of the mind and acts of God. God's ways are not our ways. Our minds are not capable of understanding Him, only catching glimpses.

I was in a professional meeting with a bright young man who was sharing insights on his conversion from Christianity to another belief system. When asked why, he said that he had examined many religions and "this one made the most sense to me."

It makes sense to a human mind to choose what is the most understandable. But it is a dangerous choice. Especially since compared to God we are less than organisms on a microscopic slide in our ability to comprehend His mind and ways.

I am convinced that the more comfortable you are with mystery, the more peace you will know in your journey here on earth.

Chad and I live under the mystery.

As Chad's mother, I have the gift and awesome responsibility of interpreting his life to him. All parents either consciously or unconsciously do this with their children. When your child has a significant disability and will not fit into the dog-eat-dog frenzied pace of our society, it is particularly needful to impart to that child a meaning larger than what he will experience in this life. Career and family and position and title and material possessions – these are not going to be the defaults in Chad's life. A gift in the brown paper bag in the situation is that life can interpreted in a way that both you and your child find joy, contentment and purpose living under God's mystery.

> "In the here and now, we must be content to live with questions only heaven will explain, trusting in the meantime that God is working out His eternal purposes beneath an intricate tapestry of mystery." [5]

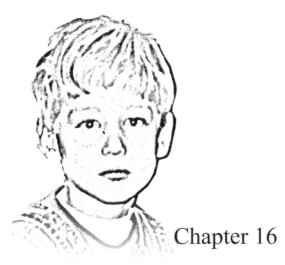

# Chapter 16

# *A Mother's Heart*

What can I say to those of you in a situation like mine? What words can I share to keep your heart alive as you journey through perilous times so you will not give up? When the world is quiet and sleeps and your heart is so weary and heavy that you cannot?

Questions bombard; your heart, mind and soul come under enemy attack. Why did this happen? What is the purpose? How on earth can I do this? What is going to happen to my child? How do I survive?

I am your sister in heart and though I do not know you personally, as I write these words I know your pain, your fear, your hopelessness.

What can I say to encourage you if you are new to the journey or bitter from the journey?

I don't know that I can, but I would like to try.

This book has been in the making for twenty six years. Actually sixty two, as my life has been one of preparation for a child with disabilities since I was born.

As my lifeline to you, may I share some perhaps much needed hope? Make a cuppa joe or hot tea or ice down a diet soda. Sugar would be good. A million years from now, you are not going to be fretting about those extra calories! What's a little cellulite between friends?

I have glorious news for you! Your pain and that of your child can be time-limited.

Read on.

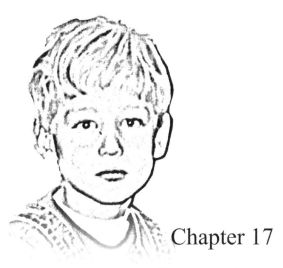

# Chapter 17

# *Someday...*

I have always had a heart for heaven. I don't ever recall a fear of death, just a fascination with and desire for heaven.

My first close experience with death was my father's. I worshiped the ground he walked on. From toddler days forward I was his appendage. My second memory, the first being my older siblings and I about aged three fleeing under a bed to escape my senile grandmother's broom, was standing on the front seat of the old '53 Chevy tucked behind my father's strong and protective shoulder as we drove into town.

Daddy was almost forty when he met Mom, a twenty-seven year old school teacher on an Indian reservation in Wisconsin. She had come to teach Bible School in several churches in central Minnesota, one being the one Daddy attended. She states she was not much taken with him until she heard him pray. In very atypical fashion for almost seventy years ago and her shy personality, upon return to Wisconsin it appears Mom was the aggressor. She began the correspondence. Daddy, happy to reciprocate, sent a picture of himself with one of his horses. Her dad thought it was a nice horse.

In October of that year, Daddy visited Mom in Wisconsin for the weekend. They were both ill for most of the weekend. She came to Minnesota for Thanksgiving. They were married on December 8, the third weekend they spent together. While she often told us she wouldn't recommend such a whirlwind courtship for us, it worked!!

In fifteen years, there were seven little ones in the busy family! In the seventeenth year of marriage, Daddy had a debilitating stroke, suffering massive brain damage, aphasia, paralysis, seizures and many other health issues and personality changes. In a moment my strong farmer-tanned dad became a pallid wizened old man.

I remember Mom packing up us seven and taking us to the hospital about ten days after Daddy's stroke. She told us that he'd look different but there is no way to prepare children for such a change. We sat in the waiting room and after a while Mom came pushing a wheelchair with an old grey-haired ashen man with a sagging mouth that drooled, his right hand with bluish fingers curled up all weird and hanging in his lap. I only remember that love was more powerful than shock and revulsion and I ran to the old man, threw myself in the wheelchair and kissed his cold cheeks. I tried not to cry and said, "DADDY I LOVE YOU!!!!" and he looked at me with sad and dazed eyes and gurgled an unintelligible sound.

We tried to be brave on the way home for Mom. But each scattered to a place of retreat when the car rolled to a stop in the driveway. I found refuge in the barn and sobbed until I thought I'd break in half--for the unfathomable loss of the safety of my father's strong arms, knowing I would never again hear the words "I love you" from the one I loved most in the world.

He lived with us until he died four and a half years later - the first day of my junior year of high school.

Although he wasn't well, I was shocked when it happened. And the seed of hope I'd nursed in my heart that somehow the Bible verses about healing would become reality, was dealt a swift and deadly blow.

Daddy had been very proud of his kids and took pride in bragging and taking credit for our meager and infrequent accomplishments. He was especially proud when we three girls sang - and called us "The Lemon Sisters". We only sang at church and often chose one of his favorite Swedish hymns.

As funeral preparations got under way, Bonnie, Meg and I decided we should sing a song at the end of the service. It would have to be *Trygarre Kan Ingen Vara (Children of the Heavenly Father)*.[6]

I was devastated at the funeral. I remember my older brother, Andy, glaring at me during the service because I was crying so hard it seemed to shake the pew, which was solid oak, bolted down and holding eight people. I weighed ninety-six pounds. I remember gaining my composure to make it through the five verses of the song, thankful we were singing in Swedish so I didn't have to really think about the words.

I was livid at everyone going down into the church basement after the burial and eating and drinking coffee and talking and, yes, laughing. I was so angry I refused to eat or drink anything. Instead I went back into the sanctuary and looked out the window overlooking the cemetery and watched Daddy being covered up with dirt and wondered how anyone could live through such pain. Or why they would want to.

But in that moment I realized I had an investment in heaven. One that was real; tangible. And with each shovel of dirt, I cried, "Daddy...Someday...."

Since then I have not only been tender for heaven. I have yearned to be there. My siblings joke about how when I go to a funeral I'm jealous of the one in the casket.

What is this, I ask myself, this deep longing for heaven?

85

Yes, it's Jesus. Yes, it's Daddy. But the heart of my longing is just an overwhelming desire to be home. HOME!!! I really don't fit in this world; I never have. I have always been a stranger, a square peg in a round hole. Those of us who march to a Different Drummer, who have chosen to take the Road Less Traveled, who have chosen God's way, don't fit. It's lonely and incredibly hard in this life. Shockingly, harder the older I get. I just want to be home - with my Father, with my family, in my own home. I want to be what I was meant to be. I want to develop my gifts and abilities that I know God has given me but have never had a chance in this life to develop. I want to have time to really get to know and be known by the wonderful people that will be my family and share my home. I want my own precious children safe and out of this icky world. And one thing I look forward to almost most of all is to meet Chad.

I want to know my son.

I don't know him. I can't know him. Autism separates us. I carried him in my body, felt him move, and loved him passionately before he saw the light of day. Then he came and was put on my chest while still connected to me, and I loved totally and forever this child. I brought him home from the hospital and held him in the darkness, watching the snow fall, the house quiet except for the sound of my rocking chair, Chad's little hand on my chest as he nursed. And I loved him beyond words. As the hot summer breeze blew through the window and I listened to the night sounds, still I rocked my nursing son in the quiet of night and thought my heart would break for the love I had for him and for the anticipation of knowing him.

But it was not to be. I had given him birth. But I could not give him life. Autism blurs who he is and the greatest heartbreak is not to know this precious little one that I hold in my heart and my arms.

But that will change! Because of Jesus! Because of heaven! I will get to know Chad.

I remember the first severely disabled person I'd ever seen. We went to a little country church and once in a while on a Sunday evening a couple would come with their teenage son. He was profoundly retarded. We didn't use terms like "developmentally delayed" in those days. He was physically mature, tall, and with lots of dark hair. I remember how the womenfolk would comment on his beautiful hair. And I marveled that they could find something beautiful about him, learning later that love and grace see the inside, not the outside.

His name was Eric. He had a bib, actually a diaper, because he constantly drooled. He had many seizures and looked very peculiar. We knew it was impolite to stare but we had never seen someone like him. His parents cared for him at home until sometime in his adulthood it apparently became too much for them and he was institutionalized.

Not long ago, I read he died. And my heart burst for joy for his mother. She is a Jesus follower. Someday she will die. I picture her being met with open arms by a tall, handsome man with a perfect mind and body, who will envelope her in his strong, tender arms and shout "Welcome home, Mom!" And she will run her fingers through his hair and weep for the joy of an eternity with her son.

Some sweet day I will be that mother. And Chad will be that son.

If I go first, I will be summoned by Jesus to be first in line in Heaven's birthing chamber and it will be my precious Chad. And I will hold him and love him and take him to Jesus. And then to Daddy to meet his grandson.

Or, if Chad goes first, I will burst into Heaven to be met by my perfect son. We will embrace and weep for joy. And he will take me to Jesus. And then to Daddy. And I will have eternity to get to know my son.

The story is told of Fanny Crosby, a prolific Christian songwriter who became blind at six weeks. Once a well meaning friend commented what a pity it was that along with the many gifts God had given Fanny He had not given her sight. Fanny replied that if she had been granted one wish at birth, it would have been that she was blind. Astounded, the friend inquired as to why. "Because," replied Fanny, "when I get to heaven, the first face that shall ever gladden my sight will be that of my Savior."[7]

Fanny saw what the well meaning friend hadn't. She's right, you know. Nothing but Jesus' face really matters after all.

Chad has been given a gift much like Fanny's. What God has chosen to withhold from Chad in this life will only intensify his joy in the next. From heaven's perspective he will say if he had been able to choose one thing in his life, it would have been that he was autistic.

So while my heart breaks in this life my joy is unparalleled. I will yet know my son.

Thanks to heaven.

Thanks to Jesus.

> He will wipe every tear from their eyes. There will be no more death or mourning or crying or pain, for the old order of things has passed away...They will see his face, and his name will be on their foreheads. There will be no more night. They will not need the light of a lamp or the light of the sun, for the Lord God will give them light. And they will reign for ever and ever. (Revelation 21:4; 22:4-5 NIV)

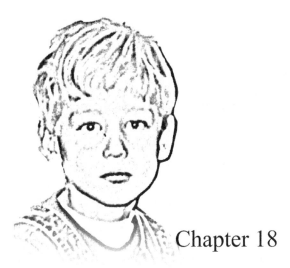

## Chapter 18

# *Treasures of Darkness*

Sometimes life is dark. You hear your name being called. You turn quickly and before you have a chance to raise your hands to protect your face, a ball whacks you squarely in the kisser.

Sometimes it's a medicine ball.

Mine was a medicine ball of autism.

I was caught off guard. Darkness was in my face.

What is the meaning of this darkness that foists itself upon me without my invitation? What is my heart to do with it? And what is *your* heart to do with *your* darkness? It may not be autism, but you have your own darkness.

Can darkness be a treasure?

It may surprise you to hear that God says "yes". Listen to *Him*, not me. He says, "I will give you the treasures of darkness, riches stored in secret places...." (Isaiah 45:3a NIV).

It's an incredible promise and even more amazing that it was made by name to a Persian king one hundred years before he was born, which is a pretty convincing argument to me that my role in God's cosmic drama is well thought out and perfectly timed. Even the dark experiences are part of the drama; maybe, *especially* the dark experiences.

I don't expect to understand all of God's ways and purposes in this life. That I settled long ago. But even this side of eternity I can see much of the wisdom of God in bringing darkness into my life.

Not only have I come to see my life and Chad's in the truth of the Cosmic Drama, I have learned the mercy of the Big Picture. Sometimes God lets us sit in darkness; requires us to sit in darkness. There is no light to move forward. It is because He loves us; because the Big Picture has something better.

I think of the Bible story of Lazarus and his two sisters, Martha and Mary, quite possibly some of Jesus' closest friends. Laz gets ill. Obviously, deathly ill as his sisters sent an unnamed but trustworthy friend to Jesus in another part of the country. This faithful ambassador told Jesus that the one He loved was sick with Jesus telling the ambassador that the purpose of the sickness was that God would be glorified.

The next two sentences in the story are riveting. "Now Jesus loved Martha and her sister and Lazarus. So, when He heard that he was sick, He stayed two days longer in the place where He was." (John 11: 5-6 NKJV)

"Now Jesus loved....so he stayed two days longer." Did I read that correctly? He loved so He stayed away? That's what it says.

Because He loved them, He did not go to them and change the horrible situation they were in. He stayed where He was, the sisters watched their beloved brother suffer and die; knowing Jesus could have come if He chose to. But He didn't. He did not intervene. Jesus let them walk in darkness because He both wrote and starred in the next act of the Cosmic Drama.

The Big Picture brought the resurrection of their brother, a far greater treasure to them, and to us, than temporary wellness of Laz.

The treasure of darkness is confusing because it is not packaged like treasure we long for or recognize. As I write these words it's almost Valentine's Day. There are millions of women dreaming they will receive a beautiful piece of jewelry from their Beloved. It will come in an elegant, velvet satin-lined box and when they see it, they will be mesmerized by the beauty sparking before their eyes.

So God pulls a paradox and packages His treasure quite the opposite. You wouldn't call Calvary a velvet-lined jewelry box. God packaged one of His greatest treasures in my life in a seven pound ounce bundle of autism and handed me Chad, beauty sparkling before my eyes. Just before Valentine's Day. Get the significance of the timing? I do. It's so like God to package His treasures in a way the world doesn't get.

The experiences of darkness in our lives are legion and unique. I believe they are God-ordained or God-permitted. God has reasons for the darkness. There are treasures there than cannot be found any place else; hidden riches only in the secret place of darkness where He takes us.

I want those treasures. I want those hidden riches. I want God to take me to those dark and secret places that so many avoid. No matter the cost. I want *everything* God has for me.

I have come to believe that each of us must make a decision, must drive down a stake, an unalterable stake into the sovereignty of Almighty God in our life. Is He sovereign or not? If so, He is sovereign in all and I will trust Him. There's no half-belief. Either we drive down an unmovable stake and trust the great and loving heart of God in our life, or we abandon our "faith" since it really is not a faith worth hanging on to.

Yes, darkness is hard and we will struggle with the human pain and loss that brings us into the darkness. And this we must regularly grieve by times alone with our heart, honestly pouring out before God the anguish of our heart and spirit and the unspeakable pain and devastation it wreaks on our humanity. This honesty before God is essential. And this honesty before man is an incredible witness as to our authenticity which is winsome and real and creates a God-thirst in their hearts.

As we walk together in the darkness, my Sovereign God and I, I have learned that it's not really dark in the darkness! Actually, it's LIGHT! It's just a different light. You need eyes that see a different spectrum of Light. It's like the brilliant stars that illuminate the clear Rocky Mountain skies. *Though I sit in darkness, the Lord himself will be my light. (Micah 7:8)*

Years ago, our family saw the Omni presentation "Everest". We watched in awe as climbers left their only comfort, their tents, in the black of night to make the final ascent, one small step after another, laboring for each breath. Their only light: the little bulbs on their helmets, illuminating just the next step. They were totally dependent on this light; certain death awaiting missteps.

The visual was haunting: several tiny lights lost in a vastness, headed toward an indiscernible summit. To the treasure: the top of the world.

God has called each of His followers to our own Everest—the climb of our life, up the sheer ice faces of life. But with a Guide better than the most trained Sherpa.

Like the climbers summiting Everest, much of the climbing, of necessity, is done in the darkness with just enough Light for the next step. Step after small step; laboring for each breath. Singularity of focus; headed to the top. Unlike the climbers of Everest, our summiting is a given. The Guide has given us His Word.

Pain? Of course. Unspeakable. Unbearable.

But part of the deal.

Let me be very clear. I'm not saying darkness is fun; it isn't. I'm not saying it's easy; it's unspeakably hard. But how to be pitied are those who walk through life doing everything in their power to avoid darkness or anesthetizing their hearts and positioning in defiance when darkness sets in. As it surely will for all us.

How many times during those dark and incredibly painful experiences of your life have you railed against the heavens asking "why", not believing you received an answer? Too many to count if you are like most people.

Like our moms with that yummy chocolate cake or that homemade apple pie, I have saved the best for last!

Let me finish what God's Word says about the treasure to be found in darkness for it answers that seemingly unanswerable "why" question.
> (And I will give you treasures hidden in the darkness – secret riches.) **I will do this so you may know that I am the Lord, the God of Israel, the one who calls you by name.** Isaiah 45:3)

You want to know why darkness invades your life? It is so that you may come to know, really know with all of your being, the Lord God, the One who designed you before He spoke the world into being.

The One who knows you by name. The One who planned the exact moment of your birth and death and knows everything that will happen in between. The One who knew every word that will ever come out of your mouth before you were conceived. The One who knows every hair on your head. The One who gave you all your gifts and talents. The One who gives you every heartbeat and every breath. The One who has absolute control over every cell, every molecule, every atom in His universe.

The One who wrote you into the Cosmic Drama with a role that only you could play and without which the Cosmic Drama would be incomplete.

The One who loves you so much He died in your place so you would not have to be held accountable for your own sin. The One who has planned a future for you so incredibly amazing and fulfilling that you cannot even dream of anything so awesome.

The One who loves you so much He will do anything to win your heart, even if it means temporary pain.

I have chosen to walk though the darkness of this life with a new vision, one that cuts through the darkness and reveals hidden treasure and secret riches. My precious son, Chad, has chosen the same. We will make it through this life, he and I. Oh, we will cross the finish line bloody and staggering and battle-scarred. It won't be pretty. But Jesus will be there - just waiting for us less than one nanosecond into eternity.

And then with a beginning so glorious there are no words to describe, Chad Timothy Brenden, God's Valiant and Faithful Warrior, will become all that God has planned for him to be for all of eternity.

*It was an honor to share my story with you.*
*Thank you for reading it. I pray for God's*
*blessings and peace upon your hard journey.*

*Best Regards,*
*Sally Brenden*

It would be an honor to have you visit us at
**www.brendenbooks.com**.

# NOTES

## CHAPTER 1: "I COULD LIVE IN SHEBOYGAN"

1. Emily Perl Kingsley, "Welcome to Holland", 1987, All Rights Reserved.

## CHAPTER 7: BORN TO LOVE GOD

2. "After 11 Years, Technique Gives Autistic Boy Voice", *St. Cloud Times,* 13 March 1992, p. 1A, 12A. "Autistic Teen Wants to Educate", *St. Cloud Times*, 13 June 1993, p. 1A.

3. http://www.rci.rutgers.edu/~lcrew/joyanyway/joy232.html

## CHAPTER 9: "I KEEP DREAMING OF THINGS TO GET EASIER"

4. Shepherd Boy, Words and Music by Raymond H. Boltz and Seven A. Millikan, 1989, Shepherd Boy ASCAP and Gaither Music Co ASCAP

## CHAPTER 15: LIVING UNDER THE MYSTERY

5. Stacy and Paula Rinehart, *Living in Light of Eternity*, (NAVPRESS, 1986), 141.

## CHAPTER 17: SOMEDAY ...

6. Trygarre Kan Ingen Vara (Children of the Heavenly Father), Lina Sandell, 1855. Translated Oskar Ahnfelt, 1872

7. http://www.christianitytoday.com/ch/131christians/poets/crosby.html

OTHER BOOKS BY AUTHOR

**AN HONORING DEATH: A Primer for Families**

Join me, a novice to death, as I direct and record my sweet Mama's three week drama of death. Walk with our family through the gut wrenching natural death process dictated by her health care directive and learn how to apply this to your upcoming situations with love, unity, and faith. Project yourself into our true story and "try on" how your family could survive and thrive in a similar and inevitable crisis. Insightful and well established hospice and palliative care explanations are added by my sister, a palliative care nurse and hospice educator, who coached us from across the country.

From the honest and intimate pre-death conversations, to Mom's re-created dining room set and her autistic grandson leading the call to worship at the memorial service, you will gain creative ideas as well as be challenged to step out of the box and confidently weave your family experience into a uniquely honoring death for your loved one.

By the way, we saved 65% over average purchased funeral services.


**GOD IN THE SERENDIPITY**
Stories for Your Heart

While most of my life, and probably yours, is lived Under the Mystery, there are cherished moments of serendipity when the Creator of the Universe surprises and overwhelms me by entering my small world. I call these glorious times, God in the Serendipity.

Special moments and unexplainable experiences when God surprises me with an awareness of His presence, power, protection, love, even tasking me to conduct Royal Business in His behalf – life changing experiences where I know in my heart of hearts it is Him.

Does He enter the lives of ordinary people living ordinary lives? Are there moments when He is so present you have no doubt that it could only be Him or do you live out your days in this customer unfriendly world of ours not convinced He has shown up for your life?

Do I have stories to tell you!

**SLIGHTLY ASKEW**
Stories for Your Heart

I serve as a warning to others.

It appears that I have been blessed with overactive stupid genes since I have been doing witless things pretty much since birth. And the sorry truth is that adulthood with its passages into career, marriage and parenthood has only added fuel to the flame.

Some experiences are so shockingly embarrassing, so totally mortifying, so absolutely foolhardy, so utterly harebrained, you really do have an obligation to humanity to share them.

Take a gander at some of mine!

(Don't be so puffed up with vainglory! Like you're perfect?!)


**MOTHERHOOD FOR TRUTHFUL WOMEN**

Not all that many decades ago, I left my professional job and became a stay-at-home Mommy for six years during what I call "Lambing Season". I went from excellence in managing people and millions of dollars to the baffling world of wee ones, one of whom would be diagnosed with autism.

I was a loving Mommy but I was an absolute "flop" at everything else related to "homemaking". I chose to embrace my deficiencies and in so doing, discovered a strange but noble calling – that of making other women feel normal, nay superior.

Lambing Season is over for me, but perhaps yours is just beginning or you find yourself in the thick of the fray. Any mother who acts as though she and her kids are perfect is lying through her teeth. And any woman who throws away her one crazy wonderful life on keeping her house spotless, should have her head examined.

## BREADCRUMBS ALONG THE PATH OF LIFE

Hansel and Gretel would have been dead meat early on had not Hansel had the wisdom and foresight to sacrifice his measly piece of bread to leave breadcrumbs along the path so they could find their way home.

The woods of life are dark and deep. Dangers lurk; peril abounds. At times my heart races at near panic. How will I ever find my way out of this impenetrable and unending forest?

Chances are you've been lost, too. But take heart. Feel the panic subside. There is a full moon rising and if you look closely, you can make out breadcrumbs along your path.

I know these woods. Let me help you get you started on the path Home.

Made in United States
North Haven, CT
23 January 2022

15154135R00059

# Resources

**Diseases**
American Heart Association https://www.heart.org
Basal Cell Carcinoma https://cancer.ca/en/cancer-information/cancer-types/skin-non-melanoma
Breast Cancer https://cancer.ca/en/cancer-information/cancer-types/breast
Canadian Cancer Society https://cancer.ca/en
Cardiovascular Disease https://www.heart.org/
Hodgkin's Lymphoma https://cancer.ca/en/cancer-information/cancer-types/hodgkin-lymphoma
Osteoporosis Disease  https://osteoporosis.ca/what-is-osteoporosis/
Vulvar Cancer https://cancer.ca/en/cancer-information/cancer-types/vulvar

**Support Groups**
Breast Cancer Support Groups https://cbcn.ca/en/abou
Cancer Patient Support https://cancer.ca/en/living-with-cancer/helping-someone-with-cancer/how-you-can-help-some-one-with-cancer
Heart Failure Support Groups https://ourhearthub.ca/patient-sup-ports/
Lymphoma Support Groups https://www.lymphoma.ca/resources/support/support-groups/
Melanoma and Basal Cell Carcinoma Support Groups https://melanomacanada.ca/support-and-resources/melanoma-skin-cancer-support-group/
Melanoma and Basal Cell Carcinoma Support and Resources https://melanomacanada.ca/support-   and-resources/
Osteoporosis Support https://osteoporosis.ca/get-support/

www.ingramcontent.com/pod-product-compliance
Lightning Source LLC
Jackson TN
JSHW040935100825
89114JS00007B/9